DEVELOPING
A NEW HEART
THROUGH NUTRITION AND
A NEW LIFESTYLE

by

Bernard Jensen, Ph.D.
Clinical Nutritionist

PUBLISHED BY:

Bernard Jensen, Ph.D.
24360 Old Wagon Road
Escondido, CA 92027 USA

First Edition

BERNARD JENSEN, Publisher
24360 Old Wagon Road
Escondido, CA 92027 USA

ISBN 0-932615-33-3

CAPTION FOR DRAWING ON INSIDE FRONT COVER: **Diagram of Lymphatic & Blood Circulation**. *Lymph fluid is derived from blood plasma that filters from blood vessels into the tissues, then finds its way into lymph vessels. Its main job is to return proteins to the bloodstream, but it also feeds tissues, gets rid of metabolic wastes and participates in the body's natural defense activities. Lymph is especially important in the feeding of tissues difficult for blood to reach, like the joints, ligaments, bones and lens of the eye. There are about 460 lymph nodes in the body, from pinhead size to as large as a bean. Undesirable bacteria and foreign matter are deposited in the lymph nodes. Lymph supplies sodium to the joints to keep them young and pliable. The body has about 40 quarts of lymph and 5 or 6 quarts of blood.*

DEDICATION

This book is dedicated to those people who are interested in growing out of and preventing heart troubles. Heart trouble is the greatest killer in the USA today, and, yet, the heart is one of the strongest organs in the human body.

CONTENTS

Dangerous? • Blood Pressure Medications. Are They Safe?
• Risk Factors in High Blood Pressure • Approaches to Reducing
Risk Factors in High Blood Pressure

From • Cereals • Dairy Products • Puddings • Sweets • Heart-Building Foods for Overweight People • Heart Tonic • The Second Heart Building Diet Period for Overweight People • Soups and Broths for Overweight People • Meat and Fish for Overweight People • Greens and Vegetables for Overweight People • The Highest Chlorine Foods • Fruit for Overweight People • Cereals for Overweight People • Drinks for Overweight People • Dairy Products for Overweight People • A Week of Heart-Friendly Menus • Guide to Herbal Seasonings • Watch for Calories in These Dressings • A Word to the Wise • Special Heart Diet—The Left-Side Diet • What Do I Mean by Starches? • Nutrition for the Heart • It Isn't Enough to Eat the Right Foods • We Must Feed the Whole Body • Walk—For Your Heart's Sake • The Importance of Brain Nutrition • Highest Sodium Foods • Highest Potassium Foods • Table of Foods Containing Heart Salts

INTRODUCTION

For over 60 years now, I have been teaching my patients secrets of the heart—ways of taking care of the heart that, until recently, seemed to be ignored or cast aside by mainstream health care professionals. I have seen wonderful recoveries by men and women from advanced levels of atherosclerosis, and even from disabling heart attacks and strokes. I have seen extreme blood pressures return to normal in as brief a time as 7 days.

How did I do this?

I taught my patients that cardiovascular health is mainly dependent on our lifestyle. I taught my patients that if they wanted to prevent or reverse cardiovascular disease, they had to take care of the 99% of the body surrounding the heart, as well as the heart itself. I taught them about diet, exercise, good bowel habits, posture, breathing, climate, altitude and getting rid of personal habits such as smoking, drug-taking and alcohol abuse. I talked about lowering their intake of fatty foods and eliminating sugar, salt and frying pans from our kitchens.

Heart disease is the No. 1 killer in the U.S. today, while in the 1800s diseases like cholera, tuberculosis, pneumonia and influenza were the big killers. What happened to make heart disease such a major threat in the 20th century?

For one thing, mass production factories in the industrial nations began to use workers in physically restricted jobs on high-speed production lines. Work stress was increased and physical activity was decreased. The invention of the automobile and the radio reduced physical exercise even more by promoting "sit-down" transportation and recreation. Since the 1950s, television has further crippled our nation's motivation to exercise, and the family farm has given away to agribusiness, large-scale farming done with big machines. Now our food is also mass-produced. The 1980s introduced personal computers and robotics in industry. Americans, these days, spend more time sitting down than people in any other nation at any other time in history.

SINS OF CIVILIZATION

Be careful of the five sins of civilization, which include, **wheat** (obesity cause), **sugar** (acid forming), **milk** (catarrh forming), **salt** (brings on hardening in the arteries and sodium imbalances), **fats** (develops cholesterol). Each of these five sins is not natural foods, and they are hard for the heart to handle.

There are other historically important changes that affect our heart health. Americans eat more packaged foods and more fast foods, which are often less nutritious than home-prepared meals, when done right. They eat too much salt, sugar and fat, too little of the fiber foods. Americans worry more, owe more money and get more divorces in the last half of the 20th century than they ever did before. We live in an age of fast living, high stress, high taxes and pollution. This is all hard on the heart.

Today, conventional health science is talking about lifestyle diseases, diet and the adverse effects of smoking, alcohol abuse and drug abuse. This shows progress, but there is still some catching up to do. There are still important heart/health care guidelines being ignored or neglected by those trained in mainstream Western medical schools.

The importance of nutrition has not yet been properly emphasized in American medical schools. The relation of bowel care and bowel transit time to health and disease has been ignored by all but a handful of persons such as Dr. Denis P. Burkitt of Great Britain, Dr. Renzo Romanelli of Italy and Dr. Juan Munoz of the United States. Not enough attention has been given to mental contributions to heart disease and high blood pressure.

My purpose in writing this book is to offer both the health-concerned person and the health care professional an alternative approach in the prevention and care of cardiovascular disease other than drugs or surgery. I want to make clear that I am not opposed to drugs or surgery when used under urgent or emergency conditions. But, if less invasive health options offer reasonable hope for improvement or reversal of a particular cardiovascular disease, why should they not be used first?

The day is coming when kids will be screened in preschool for possible heart disease in the future, and put on prevention programs. High cholesterol at 6 months has been linked to high adult cholesterol. Family history could identify 60% of all at-risk children. Early screening could cut adult heart disease by 40%, according to heart researchers.

CAN WE "CATCH" HEART TROUBLE?

The average person needs to realize that we don't "catch" heart disease or high blood pressure. We eat, drink and worry them into existence in our bodies over a period of many years. We have to work hard to bring cardiovascular disease into our bodies, and we can often get rid of it or bring about great improvement if we are willing to work hard to reverse it.

Even the food industry is getting the message that lifestyle and diet are real issues in peoples' lives. Diet frozen dinners are now lower in fat and salt as well as calories, and the public has responded by buying more diet frozen meals. I'm not endorsing the product, but just pointing out that the food industry will respond to our health needs if we demand more nutritious food.

You, not your doctor, are responsible for making the choices that will determine whether you prevent, develop or reverse cardiovascular disease in your body. This book will help you see what your choices are.

In my travels around the world, I found that heart troubles are found least in areas where people live a calm, undisturbed life and where there is spiritual balance, where they realize that the spiritual life is as important as physical life—exercise, eating and working. This way of life is taught in China, where they choose to walk through life that they may have time to observe and gain wisdom as they go. In this country, we run.

In India, Indonesia and Thailand, heart disease is so rare they don't even bother to keep statistics on it. We find that in most of Asia, it is not even listed in the top ten diseases. In Japan, I believe heart disease is the No. 5 killer. The diets of people in the Far East is much simpler than ours. They use a good deal of rice, fruits, vegetables and fish, and their diets are low in fat. Heart disease has only increased in Asia in times of war when emotional strain and unusual physical hardship came upon the people. It is well that we consider taking care of our heart and circulation through a prevention program promoting physical, mental and spiritual balance.

All people, in my opinion, have a genetic makeup that favors the development of certain kinds of diseases, and we can only prevent those diseases if we follow the right lifestyle. Let me explain what I mean.

Each person is born with a mixture of constitutional strengths and weaknesses. If a person has a pancreatic weakness, he may develop diabetes—unless he includes many complex carbohydrates in his diet and avoids sugar-loaded sweets for the most part, excepting fruits and a little honey or maple syrup now and then. If a person has a constitutionally weak liver, he may get hepatitis, unless he includes a lot of green leafy vegetables in his diet, gets adequate fresh air and exercise and takes proper care of his bowel. This, of course, is a simplified view. Most people have a dozen or more genetic weaknesses, varying in the level of vulnerability, and have many more strengths than weaknesses.

A few persons have such a strong constitution that they seldom develop any disease or illness, provided that they don't neglect basic health rules altogether. Others have such weak constitutions that they have to take exceptional care of themselves all of their lives, or they become ill or diseased and have great difficulty getting rid of any affliction.

Heart disease, often thought of as a man's disease, is also the No. 1 killer of women in the U.S. Women are not "constitutionally immune" from heart disease.

If you have really understood what I have just now explained about constitutional strengths and weaknesses, you will also understand how important it is to use the wholistic view in evaluating your health and physical fitness, and in designing ways to prevent or get rid of particular diseases—such as heart disease—that you may have. Because every organ in the body directly influences every other organ, gland and tissue in the body, our strategy for heart health **must include the whole body.**

When we look at the whole body, we find that it is made up of the dust of the earth, a complex arrangement of organs, glands and tissues composed of chemical elements. Every disease and disturbance causes changes in the chemical makeup of the body, and every chemical deficiency changes the structure and activity of the living cells that make up our bodies. Disease always involves chemical imbalance and chemical shortages, not only in the organ mainly affected by the disease, but in every other part of the body as well. When a lack of adequate potassium is causing heart problems, that lack exists throughout the body and is causing problems in the nerves, muscles, kidneys and many other tissues.

So, to take care of the heart, or any other organ in danger of chemical imbalance, **we have to feed the whole body. To take care of the heart, we have to supply all the chemical elements needed to strengthen all the glands, organs, systems and tissues that support the heart.** This is a very important principle to remember. We find that whenever there is one chemical deficiency, there are others. Chemical elements in the body work together, and if the body is deficient in one element, you can be sure others are missing.

The wholistic view of health looks to the whole body in evaluating the causes of disease and in seeing what needs to be done to reverse a disease. You can't reverse arteriosclerosis by only feeding the heart, exercising the heart, resting the heart and so on, while neglecting a toxic, underactive bowel. Every beneficial thing you do to build up that heart will be torn down by the toxins circulating in the blood from the underactive bowel. Those toxins pass through the heart with the blood and contaminate the heart tissue. We also have to look to the lungs for proper oxygenation, the thyroid to keep up the metabolism and the medulla to regulate important heart functions.

You can see, then, that we must take care of the underactive bowel and every other malfunctioning organ if we want to bring up the health level of the heart. It will help to view the body as a **community** of organs, glands and tissues, each one either helping or hindering all the others. We can help the community best by turning the hindering organs into helping organs. What is the best way to accomplish this? Often it is by raising the health level of the community as a whole.

I want to mention here that the current approach to heart disease which calls for drastic reductions in sodium intake must be regarded with both caution and wisdom. Every cell in the body needs a certain amount of sodium to live and function. The stomach, bowel, joints and lymphatic system cannot do their jobs without an adequate amount of sodium. Nerve impulses cannot travel from one nerve to another unless there is both sodium and potassium to assist the impulse in crossing the gap between nerves.

So, if we cut back too much on sodium, we harm the body as a whole while trying to help the heart in particular. The result can be indigestion, poor bowel function, over-acidity in the body, irritated nerves and stiff joints.

We will talk more about salt later in this book, but I must say that we should avoid table salt and get our sodium mainly from the natural form of it in vegetables and fruits. Table salt is an inorganic chemical, almost as powerful as a drug, and should be avoided. It has the wrong kind of sodium. The right kind of sodium is bonded to complex molecules in our foods and is assimilated and used differently in the body. We need to learn to think right to use sodium properly.

NEW GUIDELINES FOR HEART
TESTS AND THERAPIES

The American Heart Association, the American College of Cardiology and the American College of Physicians recently published voluntary guidelines for doctors and hospitals aimed at protecting patients from unnecessary tests for heart disease and from inexperienced doctors. The guidelines describe the kind of training, education and experience doctors should have before they are allowed to perform angioplasty, which opens up clogged arteries; echocardiography, which makes a sound-wave picture of the heart; and blood-flow monitoring, which measures how much blood is pumped by the heart and the pressure in arteries and veins. Over two million of these three procedures are done every year, some of them unnecessary, according to American Heart Association president, Dr. Francois Abboud.

ARTIFICIAL HEARTS AND HEART TRANSPLANTS

Finally, this introduction would be incomplete without mention of the very important pioneering attempts in our time to replace hopelessly diseased or flawed hearts with artificial hearts and heart transplants. I feel the effort to grant people with virtually untreatable heart conditions a few more years is nothing less than heroic. I am awed by the technology invested in artificial hearts and the advances in cardiology that make heart transplants possible. I have written articles about Barney Clark, the first man to be on an artificial heart, and I greatly admired his courage. But, I also feel that the greatest advance that could possibly be made in heart disease in our time would be education of the public concerning the connection between lifestyle and heart health.

If everyone in the healing arts, the news media and the government would agree to emphasize that right food habits and right living habits will prevent nearly all heart disease, we could wipe out this dreaded killer in a single generation. Nearly all kinds of heart disease can be prevented or greatly helped by changing our diet and lifestyle, but it would take 10-to-20 years of public education.

This little book is my contribution to that worthy cause.

A STATEMENT BY DR. BERNARD JENSEN

I might mention that I am not a heart specialist. I feel, sometimes, that a heart specialist is at a disadvantage in overcoming heart troubles because he knows all about the heart but does not know enough about how the rest of the body interacts with and supports the heart in times of need or distress. Good digestion is very necessary for a good working heart. Good elimination is a necessity for a good working heart. The pancreas, adrenals and thyroid are all endocrine glands that have to be as healthy as possible to have a good working heart.

Everyone has constitutional weaknesses in some of their organs, glands or tissues. Constitutional weaknesses act to make nutrient intake slower and waste elimination less efficient. When an organ does not work properly, it can affect, and be affected by, other organs. It could be toxic laden, which usually goes along with inherent weaknesses, and that organ may not be fed properly. So, these three things—inherent weakness, toxic-laden tissue and inadequate nourishment—can keep any one organ in a weak state of affairs. This can also be true of the heart. While I have not been a heart specialist, I have seen evidence that blood pressure, arteriosclerosis and hypercholesterolemia may return to normal when the whole body has been taken care of.

While the purpose of this book is to teach you how to make your heart the strongest, longest-living organ in the body, I want to make clear that I feel medical science has done wonders when it comes to heart transplants, by-pass surgery, pacemaker implants and other corrective procedures; but the heart specialist cannot afford to neglect the rest of the body and its support of various heart functions. The key to longevity and a healthy heart requires taking care of the whole person.

CHAPTER 1

GETTING TO THE HEART
OF THE PROBLEM

Every year a million-and-a-half people in the United States have heart attacks. Over 30,000 people under 55 die of heart attacks every year and nearly half-a-million people die of heart disease every year. Another four hundred thousand have strokes, which are similar to heart attacks in cause and onset, but differ by taking place in the brain. Heart attacks, strokes and other related diseases that I will discuss in this book all fall under the general name of **cardiovascular disease**.

Cardiovascular disease is the No. 1 cause of death in the United States, and my main reason for writing this book is to show you how a few simple and sensible changes in your lifestyle can strengthen your heart and lengthen your life.

Researchers call **cardiovascular disease** a "lifestyle disease." That means the development of this disease depends on what you eat, what you do, how you think and how you feel. The earlier high risk people are identified and treated, the more effective we can be against heart disease. Even children at risk for heart disease can often be identified and treated.

One of the reasons why our heart and circulatory system is so vulnerable to disease and breakdown is that it is affected by so many different events and processes. The heart is a muscle, and like other muscles, it can be overworked, strained and damaged. Unlike other muscles, it can never rest—except between heartbeats. Our circulatory system, which carries food and oxygen to every organ, gland and tissue, is like a plumbing system. Its "pipes" can get cluttered up with fat deposits on the walls or they can burst. When blood vessels are narrowed by deposits on the walls, the organs and tissues downstream from the constriction may not get as much oxygen and food as they need. When blood pressure is increased and the blood vessel walls are thin in places, the weakest area may burst.

Overwork, fatigue, high blood pressure, fatty deposits on arteries, inadequate nutrition, poor oxygenation, interference with nerve supply, glandular imbalance, toxins in the blood, lack of exercise and many other things can contribute to cardiovascular disease. Odd symptoms, like hair in the ears or a crease in the lobe of a person's ear, may be early warning signs of heart disease.

WHAT IS A HEART ATTACK?

When a heart artery becomes partly or completely blocked, a heart attack (myocardial infarction) occurs. This results in the death of those parts of the heart muscle that are deprived of oxygen. Without oxygen, tissue in any part of the body cannot survive more than a few minutes. Blockage of the blood supply to part of the brain is called a stroke, which causes death of brain tissue, just as a heart attack causes death of heart tissue.

A recent study of the effects of cocaine on the heart, conducted at Southwestern Medical Center at the University of Texas in Dallas, showed that as little as 150 milligrams of cocaine caused constriction of the arteries and reduced blood flow to the heart by 15-20 percent. It also increased the heart rate and blood pressure by 10-15 percent. This indicates that the usual cocaine user's dose of one-half-to-two grams of cocaine could cause a heart attack and sudden death.

Heart attacks and strokes together cause about a million deaths per year in the U.S. The main cause of both is a vascular disease called atherosclerosis, a disease that eventually closes off blood vessels and blocks the flow of blood. Atherosclerosis is sometimes called hardening of the arteries.

The most popular approach to dealing with blocked heart arteries is the bypass operation performed by heart surgeons. There is big money in heart operations, according to a survey of medical doctor's incomes in the late 1980s. A heart surgeon averaged over $383,000 per year, while a family doctor averaged $100,000. I don't have to tell you that heart operations are not cheap. That's another good reason to focus on prevention and not treatment at an advanced stage of the disease.

Atherosclerosis starts with damage around the edges of cells that make up the inner walls of arteries. The damaged area becomes coated with calcium. As blood flows past the rough surface of the calcium deposit, fatty deposits accumulate, forming an increasingly thick layer called plaque. Over a period of years, the plaque may cause loss of elasticity in artery walls throughout the body (hardening of the arteries) and narrowing the arterial space the blood normally flows through to get to various organs and tissues in the body. The veins and capillaries that carry blood back to the heart are not affected by hardening.

By the age of 20, the average American male has 20% blockage of his coronary arteries. This same percentage of blockage develops in the average American female at age 30, due to partial protection by female hormones.

Arteries most subject to hardening and narrowing are the large arteries: the aorta, coronary arteries, the arteries that feed the brain and the arteries that feed the kidneys. It is possible for arteries to develop fatty buildup in some parts of the bodies faster than others.

Heart attacks may happen in three ways.

Blood that is being pushed through a narrow, mostly blocked artery may form a clot and plug up the passage completely. This is called a thrombosis. A thrombosis is a heart artery clot. Thrombosis is the most common type of heart attack. An aspirin-a-day has been recommended to reduce the risk of heart attack. They say aspirin prevents blood platelets from sticking together and forming a clot. However, people with high blood pressure who take aspirin are in much greater danger of stroke due to the risk of increased bleeding. Diabetics who take aspirin regularly increase their risk of blindness from bleeding of their retina. So, always consult with your doctor before using aspirin or any other drug that interferes with blood clotting.

HEART ATTACK RISK CHART

Highest risk factors for heart attack are listed below.

- ♥ **Male and over 51 years old. (Females over 51 have half the risk of males.)**
- ♥ **Parents, brothers or sisters who have had a heart attack, stroke or heart bypass surgery.**
- ♥ **Had a heart attack already.**
- ♥ **Smoke more than 24 cigarettes daily.***
- ♥ **Have high blood pressure.**
- ♥ **Have diabetes.**
- ♥ **Regularly eat red meat or fried foods daily, more than 7 eggs a week, and use butter, milk and cheese daily.**
- ♥ **Overweight.**
- ♥ **Exercise less than once a week.**
- ♥ **Often under stress.**
- ♥ **Leg cramps after walking.**

*NOTE: A survey of 7,178 men and women who were 65 and older and had no previous history of heart disease, stroke or cancer proved that smokers in that age group had double the death rate of non smokers. Smoking kills more Americans every year than cocaine, heroin, alcohol abuse, auto accidents and suicides combined.

Another way heart attacks happen is when the fatty buildup inside an artery simply chocks off the blood supply to the "downstream" tissues. The third way is when a chunk of plaque breaks off, floats down the bloodstream and plugs a narrow passage in an artery. The result is the same in either case—oxygen deprivation to "downstream" tissue and death of cells deprived of oxygen. The attack may be milk or severe, depending on how much tissue damage occurs.

When your doctor talks about arteriosclerosis, he is using the overall name for many diseases of the arteries, including hardening of the arteries. Atherosclerosis is the most often found type of arteriosclerosis, and means the same thing as hardening of the arteries. Other names for this same condition are coronary heart disease, coronary artery disease, ischemic heart disease or arteriosclerotic heart disease.

Let's look at a few other important cardiovascular conditions.

STROKE AND ITS EFFECTS

Stroke is similar to a heart attack but happens in the brain. More than 400,000 people have a stroke each year in the U.S. This condition, also called cerebrovascular accident, is a sudden blockage of oxygen to some part of the brain. Strokes occur suddenly, and the damage they cause in the brain usually results in some kind of physical disability (such as loss or impairment of speech), mental disability (such as loss of memory) or both.

There are three main types of strokes. The most common, cerebral thrombosis, is caused by a clot that forms within the blood vessel walls. A clot that forms elsewhere in the body and travels into the brain to cause a blockage is called a cerebral embolism. A third type of stroke is cerebral hemorrhage, caused by a burst blood vessel.

The most dangerous risk factor for stroke is high blood pressure, which increases risk by seven times. Other risk factors include a fatty diet, lack of exercise, alcohol and cigarettes.

Women who take estrogen-based birth control pills are also at risk, and the particular risk is significantly increased for smokers.

ANGINA PECTORIS—CHEST PAINS

When hardening of the arteries has reached a degree of blockage that allows only a barely adequate amount of blood to get to the heart, any physical activity excess (such as running upstairs) causes a lack of oxygen to the overtaxed heart. The result is chest pain, often accompanied by a feeling of suffocation. Sometimes the pain runs down the left shoulder, arm and hand.

Angina pectoris is not a disease, but a symptom of either hardening of the arteries or of coronary artery spasms.

Angina can be reversed in some cases if you are willing to work to reverse the blockage by using an extreme low fat diet, such as the Pritikin diet, and make other lifestyle changes. Management of angina can also be done at easier levels, as follows:

♥ Avoid emotional stress
♥ Reduce physical exertion
♥ Eat 5 small meals instead of 3 larger meals
♥ Get rid of any excess weight
♥ Stop smoking
♥ Follow your doctor's advice.

SALT

It has been said that the average person consumes about half an ounce of salt daily. This is usually more than adequate, but in extreme heat when perspiration is heavy, more than the usual amount of salt is lost from the body and a deficiency can result. It is characterized by weakness, cramp-like pains and nausea.

There have been many experiments with people who perspire heavily, and when they are given salt water, they just seem to come right back.

We find it is necessary to replace the salt that we are losing daily through perspiration. The problem is, we don't always put enough salt back into the body. Or, we don't put back the right kind. We use common sodium chloride (table salt), and we find that this kind of salt has undesirable side effects. This is what we have to be careful about. It is claimed that there are about 3 ounces of salt present in the body of an adult at any one time, and the elimination of salt is regulated by the outer layer of the adrenal gland.

The human body also uses salt to provide chlorine required to synthesize hydrochloric acid. This is a significant digestive substance secreted by the stomach. Pepsin performs its digestive function only in the presence of hydrochloric acid. We find here that the stomach wall has to have a reserve of sodium in that stomach wall in order to have the proper protection from the hydrochloric acid secreted.

We find that the excessive salt in the diet can affect the kidneys and blood pressure adversely. A low salt or salt-free diet is prescribed in such cases. When we have problems with the kidneys and low blood pressure, we also have to supply the chemical elements that are needed for repair and correction, which can only come from foods.

It is also claimed that if we could just reduce the amount of salt we take into the body from half an ounce to 1/10th ounce, it may work to reduce edema, swelling due to excess water. There are many people who hold water, and sodium has an affinity for water that causes us to hold more water in our systems. This is especially so if we use an excess amount of salt in our diet. Because of this, water can accumulate in the tissues, and of course this shows the imbalance of the chemical elements needed for the body. It is possibly this feature of water-holding by sodium that makes it a risk factor for high blood pressure and by heart disease.

We find that sodium chloride is also used in many medical functions. Saline solution is given intravenously when fluid has been lost by the body in bleeding and must be replaced.

HIGH BLOOD PRESSURE

High blood pressure, often called hypertension, afflicts one in six adults in the U.S. It goes hand-in-hand with hardening of the arteries and increase the risk of stroke and heart attack.

Blood pressure reading is made up of two separate figures, such as 120/70, representing the amount of pressure (in millimeters of mercury) of two different phases of heart "pumping" activity. The higher number, called the systolic blood pressure, represents the pressure in the arteries when the heart muscle contracts, pushing the blood out. The lower number of the two is the diastolic pressure, representing the relaxation phase between heartbeats.

Normal blood pressure in young adults ranges between 110 and 140 (systolic) and between 70 and 90 (diastolic). When the diastolic pressure is from 90-104, a person is said to have mild hypertension. From 105 to 120 diastolic, the condition is described as moderate-to-excessive hypertension.

Statistics show that a young man with a blood pressure of 150/100 will have a life expectancy about 16 years less than others his age with blood pressure in the normal range.

Drugs used to treat high blood pressure include diuretics, sympatholytics and vasodilators. The problem is, all drugs have side effects, including these. Diuretics can cause breast enlargement, high blood sugar and increased uric acid levels. Some diuretics cause low potassium. Vasodilators change the heart rate, may cause water retention and can bring on a type of lupus. Sympatholytics can cause impotence, depression, diarrhea and water retention. All of these are undesirable side effects.

The cause of high blood pressure is unknown, and even the risk factors of excess sodium intake, high blood cholesterol, smoking, coffee and alcohol are not proven risk factors.

Pressure sensitive nerve ends in arterial walls sense any change in blood pressure, signaling the brain. The brain signals the arteries to dilate or constrict, adjusting the pressure toward normal. Fear and anger send the blood pressure up. Grief is said to lower blood pressure.

Whatever the cause of high blood pressure, carefully done studies show that hypertension increases the chances of heart attack, hardening of the arteries, stroke and kidney disease.

FADS AND FANCIES

Periodically, theories and treatments concerning cardiovascular disease become popular fads. Then, just as quickly, the fad turns into a fancy and fades away.

The recommendation of low sodium diets for those at risk for heart attacks and strokes must be carefully evaluated. Sodium from food is needed by the gastrointestinal system, the nerves, the joints and the lymph system. Over a period of time, sodium deficiency can bring on joint problems, indigestion, poor assimilation of nutrients, stomach ulcers, lymph congestion, nerve irritation, and excess acidity throughout the body. We need the kind of sodium that occurs naturally in fruits and vegetables. We don't need the kind that occurs in table salt, which is sodium chloride in an ionic, crystalline form, refined by heating at high temperatures and adulterated with magnesium carbonate to make the salt flow without sticking or clumping. Don't let yourself become confused. Avoid table salt (and chemical salt substitutes) and use vegetable broth seasoning instead. But, be sure to use plenty of sodium-rich foods like celery, okra, whey, strawberries, green leafy vegetables and sun-ripened fruits.

Using water softeners that take the calcium out of hard water and replace it with sodium can also increase the risk of heart attack, when the water is used for drinking. Many families have stopped using water softening units for that reason. Chemical sodium is hard on the cardiovascular system.

The Food and Nutrition Board of the National Academy of Sciences in 1980 issued a report saying that dietary cholesterol is not a problem. More recent studies have reversed that position, advising that 25% of U.S. men and 30% of U.S. women have cholesterol levels that indicate moderate-to-high risks of heart attack. Now, we are told that cholesterol is made up of good cholesterol (high-density lipoprotein or HDL) and bad cholesterol (low-density lipoprotein or VASODILATOR). High-density cholesterol is believed to protect us against heart disease, while low-density cholesterol increases the risk of heart attack. Most food cholesterol occurs in animal products—meat, eggs, butter, cheese, milk and so on. If these products are not heated over 212 degrees F., then the lecithin that normally accompanies cholesterol in food balances the cholesterol and keeps it in solution, solving the problem. Animal products high in cholesterol are acceptable as foods if not overheated, fried in grease or otherwise refined to remove or destroy the lecithin. Eggs, in my view, are one of nature's best proteins. On the other hand, I don't believe in eating eggs—or any other single food—every day.

In 1974, a book titled *Type A Behavior and Your Heart* by Drs. Meyer Friedman and Ray Rosenman became something of a controversial best seller. Friedman and Rosenman claimed that a particular type of behavior—"type-A behavior" might be at the root of all heart disease. They blamed heart disease primarily on stress caused by a particular personality/behavior characterized by aggressiveness, impatience, competition almost to the point of combativeness, urgency, hostility—in other words, ambitious, overbearing workaholics. More recent studies have found no evidence linking "type-A behavior" with heart attacks.

There are many verifiable contributing factors to heart diseases, but watch out for those that fall in the "fads and fancies" category. Not everything you find in print is reliable. Time will show whether it is or isn't. Until a particular treatment, theory or health recommendation is proven, it is best to stay with what is really known and what really works.

A CLOSE LOOK
AT PRESIDENT EISENHOWER'S HEART ATTACK

In 1955, President Dwight D. Eisenhower had a heart attack while on vacation in the Rocky Mountains of Colorado. He was in his sixties at the time, a former Supreme Commanding General of Allied Forces in Europe during World War II. He was no stranger to stress. President Eisenhower was a greatly liked president, and I followed the news of his heart attack very closely.

I think the first thing to be considered was that he took his vacation at a high altitude, where there is less oxygen. This is hard on the heart, and it takes some time for the body to adjust to the change from sea level to the high Rocky Mountains. The President loved trout fishing, and that is what attracted him to the Rockies.

For lunch, President Eisenhower had a hamburger with onions, which is often very gas-forming. The hamburger was on a white-flour bun. The doctor who checked him thought he was suffering from a little indigestion, and the President was soon over his symptoms. I believe the gas in his stomach put pressure against the heart which contributed to what followed.

The next morning, the President got up at 5 am to go trout fishing. The shock of early rising after the mild heart symptoms of the day before was compounded by what happened next.

The weather had turned uncomfortably cold, but President Eisenhower went fishing anyway. He put on his waders and struggled out into the icy water of a snow-fed stream to fly fish. Then snow began to fall. I believe the cold caused his arteries and veins to contract, increasing the load on his heart.

After returning to his cabin, instead of resting, the President had a hearty breakfast of hotcakes and syrup with fried eggs, bacon, sausage and coffee. From the sugary syrup and protein to the caffeine in the coffee, the high stimulation pushed his heart still closer to the edge. He should have had a breakfast of whole, pure, fresh and natural foods, but instead he had another gas-forming meal like the hamburger he'd eaten the day before.

When breakfast was over, the President headed for the golf course with a few friends and played 18 holes of golf. If this kind of schedule was typical of the President's lifestyle, it's a wonder he didn't have a heart attack years before! High altitude, gassy, stimulating foods, cold weather, over exertion—this is almost a recipe for heart attack. This is a positive diet and attitude that contributed to his heart attack. The yin (the positive balance) and yang (the negative balance) were not balanced as worked out in the study of Ayurvedic healing, or Chinese healing.

On September 24, 1955, heart specialist Dr. Paul Dudley White was flown to Fitzsimmons Army Hospital in Denver, Colorado, as a consultant to Major General Howard Snyder and other doctors treating President Eisenhower, who suffered a heart attack. The President pulled through, and Dr. White served as his friend and medical advisor through his recovery period.

President Dwight Eisenhower learned from his experience and later had this to say: "I must keep my weight at a proper level. I must have a short midday breather. I must normally retire at a reasonable hour, and I must eliminate many of the less important social and ceremonial activities." If he had learned this lesson on his own, and not from Dr. White, the President might not have had a heart attack.

Dr. White is my favorite doctor. During President Eisenhower's recovery, his many television and news media interviews informed our whole nation—and the people of many other countries, of the lifestyle factors that contribute to heart disease. Overnight, this kindly, wise man increased the health consciousness of many people with his discussions of the President's heart attack and recovery.

Here are some excerpts from this wise doctor's philosophy:

It is my experience...that hard work, physical or mental, never killed a healthy man.

We know a thousand times more about diseases than our predecessors did generations ago, but...infinitely less about health.

The greatest challenge of public health today is keeping the middle-aged physically fit.

I have long advocated moderate exercise as one of the best ways to keep the heart in good condition.

We must give first priority to research in preventive medicine.

In this push-button age, man is overeating and pampering himself and "the life of Riley" often leads us into a lot of early coronary disease, high blood pressure and diabetes.

Overeating may play even more of a role in the destiny of the world than the under-nutrition of hundreds of millions of representatives of the common man.

Truly, Dr. Paul Dudley White is one of the greatest men in the healing arts of our time.

CLIMATE AND THE HEART

Many years ago, I visited three places where men—at least some men—lived unusually long lives. At the University of Loja in Ecuador, I was told that people with heart trouble traveled to Vilcabamba, only 60 miles away, to get relief from their problems. So, I went there.

I met Señor Carpio, who, at the age of 129, had never seen a doctor. I found a man in his 90s, still working 10 hours a day manufacturing furniture. At 132 years of age, Señor Toledo remembered having pneumonia at the age of 110, which he survived with the aid of herbal teas. The food and lifestyle habits appeared to be the same as other places we had visited in Ecuador. But something was contributing to the health and longevity of these people, something that brought rapid recovery and improvement to visitors with cardiovascular ailments as well.

On another occasion, I traveled through Kutkey and Armenia to the Republic of Azerbaijan in the USSR, where I interviewed Mr. Shirin Gasanov, 153 years of age. His blood pressure was 130/80, his pulse rate was 75 beats per minute.

Gasanov told me, through an interpreter, that he ate mostly vegetables, fruit, kasha (buckwheat), milk products like matsoni (yogurt) and a little boiled meat once in a while. His last meal in the day was at 6 pm, a small meal, and he ate nothing after that. He drank a lot of water. The age of his youngest child was 60. Something like 70% of the people in the village were his relatives.

I heard of an older man in the area but could not get permission to see him. His name was Shirali Mislimov, whose children, grandchildren, great-grandchildren and so forth numbered 220. He had never been sick a single day in his life. His blood pressure was 125/75, his pulse rate was 72. His age at the time was 168 years.

Gasanov, Mislimov and other century-plus men in this mountainous area were shepherds in their younger days. Their diets were sparse, and walking long distances with their sheep was part of their job. I reported over 20 more Azerbaijanis over 100 years old and published their pictures and brief biographies in my book *World Keys to Health and Long Life*.

Visiting the Hunza Valley in Pakistan and being invited to stay in the Mir's palace has been one of the great highlights of my travels. Heart disease among the Hunza people was unknown at the time of my visit. The Hunzas lived in an isolated valley high in the Himalayas. I met several men over 100 years old who had all their teeth, were mentally and physically active and still worked in the fields every day. These people ate two meals a day, including raw turnips, carrots, peas, spinach, green leafy vegetables and fruits such as apples, pears, cherries, mulberries and apricots (both fruit and seed), which were dried and kept as a winter food. Their grains included millet, buckwheat, barley, rye and corn. They used very little milk and ate a small quantity of meat in the winter only. The rich soil on their terraced mountainside gardens was washed down by water melting from glaciers, and they drank mineral-rich glacier water.

In all three places: Vilcabamba, Ecuador; Azerbaijan, USSR; and Hunza Valley, Pakistan, the low incidence of cardiovascular disease and unusual longevity seemed to be related to several factors.

All three locations were in the mountains, with good soil, clean air and good drinking water. Because the majority of the people were poor, transportation was primarily by walking—the best heart exercise. For the same reason, the relative poverty of these areas, the people ate simple, locally-grown foods for the most part, and may have seemed underfed by our own standards. They had limited access to tobacco, alcohol, refined foods, packaged foods, meat, colas and other commercial soft drinks and consumer food products so common in wealthier Western nations. Underfeeding, I should say, has been found to increase longevity in laboratory animals.

The isolated, rural locations protected the local inhabitants from the stress and trauma of political and military conflicts, and their lack of access to world news undoubtedly allowed them greater peace of mind. Obviously, they were not exposed to life in the fast lane, nor the crime, economic ups and downs, and noise of more "civilized" areas. In the Hunza Valley, there were no hospitals, police stations, jails, drug stores, bars, gangs, drug dealers or even dentists, when I was there.

We can't reproduce these conditions in the United States and other Western nations, but we can—and should—learn from them.

CHAPTER 2

WHAT IS A HEALTHY HEART?

I would like to be able to say that a healthy heart is one composed of constitutionally strong tissue, with a regular beat and clean, normally-formed valves. But it is impossible to describe a healthy heart without talking about an individual's health history, dietary habits and bowel condition—among other things!

We are finding more and more young people in the U.S. with fatty deposits in their arteries—some even in their teens—due to an overly fatty food regimen. A recent physical fitness test at schools throughout the U.S. shows a decline in students' cardiovascular endurance and an increase in their weight. This is the beginning of **hardening of the arteries**. People with a history of rheumatic fever may have another heart problem—inflammation in the heart tissue that leaves the mitral and aortic valves deformed by scar tissue, unable to open or close properly. Constipation may contribute to such levels of toxins in the blood that the heart tissue is weakened after a time. There are many things that can go wrong with this essential organ.

Heart health depends on what culture you are in. The Masai tribesmen in East Africa use a high-cholesterol diet but never seem to have heart trouble. Masai herdsmen may walk 50 to 60 miles a day without strain. Masai warriors were persuaded to try a treadmill brought by a U.S. college professor. The group averaged 23 minutes on the treadmill, compared to 14 minutes for an average U.S. male college student. Their pulse rates rose but not their respiratory rates. Two of the Masai men got on the treadmill when it was set at a 30 degree incline, and they walked for 30 minutes. These people have wonderfully strong and durable hearts.

If we stop and think about it, the health of our hearts is affected by every other organ, gland and tissue of the body. In order to more fully understand what a healthy heart is, we need to understand how the heart is related to other important organs and processed in our bodies. Before I attempt to do this, I want to discuss the basic anatomy of the heart and how it works.

THE HARD-WORKING HEART

The adult human heart is a fist-sized organ weighing about two pounds, constructed like a two-story house with four rooms—two rooms upstairs (the right and left auricles) and two rooms downstairs (the right and left ventricles). Old blood enters the right auricle, depleted of oxygen and loaded with carbon dioxide waste. From the right auricle, this old blood is forced into the right ventricle directly below, from which it is pumped into the lungs by way of the pulmonary artery.

In the lungs, carbon dioxide is released and the blood is freshly oxygenated. This crimson oxygen-laden blood passes into the pulmonary veins and enters the left auricle in the second-story level of the heart. Blood from the left auricle is forced down into the left ventricle directly below. From the left ventricle, the freshly oxygenated blood is pumped into the aorta, the main artery that feeds the whole body.

From the aorta, the anterior (front) and posterior (rear) coronary arteries deliver blood to the heart muscle itself. It is the coronary arteries that so often develop a thick, hard layer of cholesterol and triglycerides, setting up the **arteriosclerosis** that eventually leads to a heart attack if not properly taken care of. (A heart attack is often called "a coronary.")

Every minute, the normal heart beats from 65 to 75 times. In a lifetime of 70 years, the heart will beat over 2-1/2 billion times, working 24 hours a day. The heart begins working before birth and only rests between beats. Otherwise, it never stops to take a break and never takes a vacation.

The heart pumps blood over 60,000 miles of blood vessels at the rate of a gallon a minute. In a lifetime, the heart may pump nearly 37 million gallons of blood. There is no man-made pump that can match the efficiency and reliability of the human heart.

We find out that besides the impressive strength and reliability of the heart, there are always signs of slowdown by the age of 30. It doesn't matter whether you are male or female, obese or slender, in good or poor physical condition. Aging always decreases endurance and exercise performance in each person, as compared to his or her abilities earlier in life. A healthy lifestyle slows both signs of aging and the reduction of the heart's efficiency but doesn't stop it. The heart's oxygen consumption and pumping capability begins to slow down at age 30, with the rate of slowdown increasing through the 40s, 50s and 60s. Researchers say this means that exercise may be more important as people get older.

In the heart itself and throughout the vascular system, one-way valves automatically open and close with each forward "push" of the blood, preventing any reverse flow or seepage. Small children have a more rapid heartbeat than that of adults.

During exercise, three or four times the usual amount of blood is pumped each minute. An athlete at peak performance may be pumping as much as nine times the normal amount of blood—over nine gallons per minute!

If you followed a single drop of blood through the entire circulatory system of the body, you would find that it circulates completely every six minutes.

THE PULSE—YOUR HEARTBEAT

Every time you go to the doctor, he or his nurse will put two fingers on your wrist and look at their watch. They are counting your pulse rate, the number of times your heart beats per minute. A healthy pulse is between 65 and 85 beats per minute. However, a marathon runner or bicycle racer who practices regularly may have a healthy pulse rate as low as 40 beats per minute. Children tend to have higher pulse rates, but a fast pulse rate can also result from chronic alcohol abuse, which injures the heart and weakens its ability to pump.

Cigarettes, coffee and appetite reduction pills will speed up the pulse. So can infection, fever, stress or pain. An overactive thyroid speeds up your pulse. An underactive thyroid slows it down.

An irregular heartbeat can be nothing important in some cases. In other cases, it can signal that your life is in danger. Only a careful examination by your doctor can determine the difference.

LOCATION OF THE HEART

In our bodies, the heart is located slightly to the left of the center of the chest. Roughly cone-shaped, the heart is about five inches long, about three-and-a-half inches wide at its widest point. The cavities are lined with a membrane called the **endocardium**, and the heart muscle itself is protected by a thin membrane called the pericardium. The wall between the left and right sides is called the septum.

The heartbeat is triggered by an electrical discharge from the **sinoatrial node** in the upper right heart chamber's muscle structure. About a thousandth of a volt is discharged, causing the contraction of the heart muscle that forces the blood from the ventricle. The rate of the heartbeat is regulated by nerves from the brain. Not only muscular activity of the body, but also emotional reactions, stress or sleep can raise or lower the heartbeat rate.

The **sinoatrial node** initiates each heart cycle, so it is called the "pacemaker." The electrical impulse triggered by this node travels over nerve fibers and interacts with a second node, the **atrioventricular node** , located between the upper right and lower right chambers of the heart.

The heart does not depend on the brain or other parts of the nervous system to make it beat. It has its own "electrical power plant" and initiates its own electrically-stimulated contractions.

KING OF THE ORGANS

Perhaps because the heart pumps blood to supply the oxygen and nutrient needs of all the organs, glands and tissues of the body, it is called the "king of the organs." The king's responsibility is to meet the needs of his subjects.

The king, of course, is also dependent upon his subjects for protection, taxes and for supplying his needs. Similarly, the heart is dependent on all other organs.

The liver detoxifies the blood and manufactures cholesterol, which, together with dietary intake of cholesterol and fats, contributes to atherosclerosis—hardening of the arteries. A healthy liver, together with a healthy, low-fat diet, helps keep the risk of cardiovascular disease down.

The bowel, although not directly related to the heart, influences cardiac health in several ways. The research of Denis Burkitt, M.D., has shown that diets rich in fiber reduce bowel transit time and may reduce the incidence of heart disease. In East Africa where natives use high-fiber diets, Burkitt found very little heart disease. Increasing the amount of fiber foods in the diet also helps prevent constipation, the main cause of toxic blood. Indole, skatole and other bowel-originated toxins have been found in the blood of constipated persons. In my experience, a reflex relationship between colon and the heart contributes to heart trouble when diverticulosis is present in the descending colon. A clean, healthy bowel with normal transit time contributes to a clean bloodstream and a healthy heart.

The kidneys filter the blood, conserve water and electrolytes such as potassium and sodium, and help control the acid-alkaline level of the blood. They also help control blood pressure. (High blood pressure is an important risk factor contributing to heart attack and stroke.) The mineral potassium is essential to healthy heart function, neutralizing metabolic acid wastes in the heart muscle. To a lesser extent, sodium is essential in maintaining the health of heart membrane and ligaments. The kind of potassium and sodium our bodies need is the kind we get from foods, not from table salt or inorganic mineral tablets.

The lungs oxygenate the blood and get rid of carbon dioxide, the breakdown product of carbonic acid waste. Oxygen is vital to every cell of the body. If oxygen intake is reduced by smoking, lack of exercise or lung damage, the whole body is impaired—but especially the heart and the brain. Smoking contributes to heart disease. (In fact, studies have shown that more smokers die of virtually every disease than nonsmokers.)

The endocrine gland system, directed by the hypothalamus of the brain, affects the heart in many ways. I describe these ways in detail in my chapter on stress, so I will only cover the highlights here. Endocrine glands can speed up the heart rate, increase oxygenation and release more blood sugar to generate strength and energy to meet emergencies. They help control the sodium-potassium balance, as regulated by the kidneys. These things affect the health of the heart, sometimes to the point of disaster. Often, we don't realize what a great effect the glands have on the body.

Because we are what we eat, the stomach and small bowel, which do most of the digesting of foods, are necessary for heart support. But, the digestive system can only do so much with a bad diet. We need to know what kinds of foods keep the heart healthy and strong.

Last, but not least, many brain centers and processes are essential to a healthy heart. I have called the heart "the king of the organs," but we have to realize that the brain is really the power behind the throne. The "chest brain," located in the medulla, has respiratory, heart and vasomotor centers that control breathing, heart activity and blood vessel diameter changes. If this is damaged, the heart is always affected. The thalamus and hypothalamus, important nerve switchboards that connect the higher brain functions (thought, feelings, memories) with motor nerves that regulate the heart and other organs, often influence heart rate and breathing. While it may not be true that the heart is the "center of love," the heart—regulated by the brain—can change dramatically when we see someone we love. It can also change a great deal when we experience negative emotions. My feeling is that the brain is the most important organ to take care of in preventing cardiovascular disease.

What we must learn—for our own survival and quality of life—is to **consider the heart as a member of a community of organs, each dependent on all the others for its health**. Yes, we have to take care of the heart. But as we do, we also need to do our best to take care of every other organ in the body, so each can do its part in keeping our heart healthy.

LOOKING AT THE WHOLE PICTURE

Since the reason for this book is to help you know how to prevent heart disease by building a healthy heart, we need to ask, "Is there such a thing as a healthy heart?" The answer is "yes and no." The answer is "no" if we consider that there is no such thing as a perfect heart. But "yes," there is such a thing as a healthy heart, and "yes," there is a way to build one.

In past years, the Japanese whose diet is low in beef and dairy products, have had a remarkably low incidence of heart disease. Fish is a regular part of their diet, and fish oils are known to counteract atherosclerosis. Heart disease is highest in countries like the United States, Denmark and New Zealand, where large amounts of beef and dairy products are consumed. Dr. Denis Burkitt found very little heart disease among East African rural tribes, who use high-fiber grains as a mainstay in their diet. Studies of Eskimo tribes in Canada and Greenland show that a high fat, high cholesterol diet doesn't necessarily lead to heart disease on its own. They are, however, physically very active. Tribes in New Guinea and in the Kalahari desert have a low incidence of heart disease.

Is aging a major factor in heart disease? Indirectly, I suppose we must answer, "yes." Bodies slow down over the years, no matter how "smart" we eat or live. We all realize that as our bodies slow down, we become more vulnerable to disease, simply because we assimilate nutrients more slowly and with greater difficulty, and we get rid of metabolic and other wastes less efficiently. Our constitutionally weak organs begin to slow down. These are facts of life. Yet, we should always do the best we can to keep ourselves healthy no matter what our age.

Look at the following chart, and you'll see some interesting body statistics that change as we age.

BODY CHANGES WITH AGING*

Age	Muscle Strength (%)	Lung Capacity (%)	Blood Cholesterol (mg/dl)	Maximum Heart Rate (%)	Kidney Function (%)
25	100	100	198	100	100
45	90	82	221	94	88
65	75	62	224	87	78
85	55	50	206	81	69

*Figures taken from **Newsweek** magazine, March 5, 1990.

In 1980, over 25 million Americans were past 65 years of age. When the body's efficiency is diminished as shown in the preceding chart, the processes that contribute to disease must be countered by a balanced diet and supplement regimen, regular exercise, a healthful lifestyle, a cheerful disposition and tissue cleansing (as described in my book *Tissue Cleansing Through Bowel Management*). To prevent disease and ailments, we must compensate as much as possible for metabolic slowdown associated with aging.

Many researchers believe that cardiovascular disease is a disease of civilization. That's something to think about.

Almost everyone is born with a healthy heart and blood vessels. Many people on the "safe end" of the alarming statistics for cardiovascular disease and mortality—that is, **those who don't acquire heart disease** but who live in the United States, have relatively healthy hearts. We can point to the Seventh Day Adventists, a religious denomination that follows a vegetarian way of life for the most part. Their mortality rates for heart disease are much lower than the national average.

The great scientist Alexis Carrel kept a thin microscope slice of chicken heart alive for 16 years by feeding it casein extracted from egg yolk. We find that proper nutrition is essential for a sound heart.

Dr. V.G. Rocine reported that a group of university professors from Sweden determined from animal experiments that the heart had several sources of energy: 1) Energy from foods; 2) cerebral and cerebellar sources of energy; 3) a source from the medulla or "chest brain"; 4) a source from the spinal cord; and 5) a source related to respiration. We realize that the nerves, brain and glands cooperate in assigning to each organ the energy it requires to do its job in the body. However, the dietetic nutrients alone can keep a thin section of heart tissue alive without the others, and I believe that a low-fat diet of whole, pure, fresh and natural foods will do more for your heart than anything else.

Vegetarianism is almost matched by regular vigorous exercise as a way of lowering the incidence of cardiovascular disease and the risk of heart attack. Women, until the age of menopause, are protected from hardening of the arteries by female hormones. As a consequence, their incidence of heart disease is low.

The key to freedom from worry about heart attack, stroke and cardiovascular disease, in general, seems to be a healthy lifestyle. We will cover the healthy heart-building lifestyle in a later chapter.

Are You A Heart Risk?

I look out over my household, my students, patients and friends all over the United States, and realize that half the people I know are having heart troubles or soon will have heart troubles. It is necessary to recognize that we must take a preventive and wholistic approach to heart health to reduce the number of heart attacks taking place every day. This is an absolute necessity if we want to live longer, healthier, more productive lives.

So, with this thought, this book is not just for the person to take care of his heart, which may have deteriorated to a degenerative stage, but rather it is for the person who wants to take care of the whole body in such a way as to include the heart. We all know that heart disease is the No. 1 killer in the USA today. So, in working for a good heart, we are using the wholistic approaches that the whole body should be built up together with the heart. This is very important!

CHAPTER 3

SYMPTOMS AND RISK FACTORS

There are many cardiovascular conditions we should be aware of besides heart attack and hardening of the arteries. Most conditions have their own symptoms. A few have no symptoms. (Some doctors say hairy ear canals, creased earlobes and bald heads are indicators of heart disease.) Heart attack and stroke often strike without warning, without any symptoms at all, but by the time you finish reading this book (or even this chapter), you should have a reasonably good idea of whether you have some degree of cardiovascular disease.

What happens when a person has a heart attack? Usually there is severe pain in the middle of the chest—some say "like an elephant sitting on my chest." There may be pains in the left arm. Breathing difficulties, heart palpitations and an ashen-gray face are often symptoms, possibly with nausea and vomiting. These are common symptoms experienced by someone who has a heart attack.

High blood cholesterol, especially a high reading of low density cholesterol, is considered an early warning signal for cardiovascular disease. An even better early warning signal may have been found by researchers from France and Israel. They say high levels of insulin in the blood may be an advance symptom of coronary heart disease. A study of 1,258 men showed that high blood levels of insulin were over three times more frequent in men with high blood pressure, obesity or glucose intolerance. Rates of heart disease were four times higher in those who had high insulin levels than the controls. High blood creatinine levels in those who already have high blood pressure signal danger from heart attack or stroke. Over 50% of the people who had both symptoms died within eight years.

Is aging a cause of heart disease? Lifestyle is more likely to be the cause, according to recent studies. Too little exercise, obesity, too much salt and too little calcium contribute to hardening of the arteries, high blood pressure and heart disease. Aging is not an automatic risk factor for heart disease.

Most cardiovascular conditions are brought on or aggravated by certain lifestyle habits. More strokes from blocked arteries happen from February to April than in other months. A few conditions are inherited, while others are of unknown origin. When some lifestyle habit like smoking, overeating or stress is known to contribute to a cardiovascular disease, it is called a "risk factor." Smoking is definitely a risk factor for several cardiovascular diseases. Cigarette smoke has almost 4,000 chemicals in it. Here are just a few newspaper article titles recently published:

Congressional Report Rips Tobacco Council

**Florida Can Sue Tobacco Firms
for Illness Costs**

"Horrible Price" Paid for Not Knowing

Tobacco Creed: Money Talks

**While Cigarette Companies Lie,
More Smokers Die**

The study that really confirmed the risk to the heart of factors that many of us in the healing arts already suspected was the Framingham Study. For 39 years, over 5,000 citizens of the town of Framingham, Massachusetts, were observed by researchers. The scientists conducting the study recorded their diets, physical activities, work and lifestyle habits. One of the risk factors pointing to heart disease was heredity, an inherited constitutional weakness in or affecting the heart. But other risk factors were things we are able to change. These included high blood cholesterol, diabetes, obesity, stress, high blood pressure, lack of exercise and smoking.

Changing even one risk factor can bring a significant reduction in risk. A University of Washington study showed that people who are physically active have half the risk that others do of suffering a first heart attack. Men who don't exercise die four or five years sooner than those who do. When other risk factors are taken care of, longevity is significantly increased.

There are unusual causes of heart disturbances that sometimes puzzle health practitioners. Bad teeth may cause infections in the body that bring on symptoms like those of heart disease. Rheumatic fever in childhood may be followed by heart trouble. A toxic thyroid condition or diverticula in the colon may cause heart disturbances. We have to be very careful how we treat the heart because so many other parts of the body affect it.

The descriptions of cardiovascular diseases, symptoms and risk factors in this chapter are designed to help you understand the range and variety of problems known to involve the heart and circulatory system. I have not attempted to make the list complete, but I believe I have covered the most important conditions. The diseases and conditions I have selected are adapted from standard medical books available to anyone, and I am in no way encouraging anyone to diagnose or treat themselves. Cardiovascular disease is a life and death matter, and if you suspect you have any of the following conditions, I urge you to see your doctor and have him give you a checkup and any tests he considers necessary.

However, you are the one who is responsible for health maintenance and prevention of disease in your body, and it is my hope that the list given here will motivate you to take better care of yourself.

CARDIOVASCULAR CONDITIONS, SYMPTOMS AND RISK FACTORS

ACUTE PERICARDITIS: Inflammation of the membrane covering the heart, possibly with fluid buildup in space between the membrane and the heart muscle.

Symptoms: Sudden chest pain, possibly reflexing to left shoulder. Pain worsens with deep breathing or coughing.

Risk Factors: Onset due to viral infection, rheumatic fever, diseases, like lupus or kidney failure.

ANEURISM: Pouching out or swelling of an arterial wall due to weakness perhaps triggered by inflammation or atherosclerosis. The danger is bursting and bleeding.

Symptoms: Depends on location and whether or not the aneurism has burst. Severe headache or unconsciousness indicates brain artery aneurism. Aorta aneurism may be signaled by chest pain, cough, difficulty swallowing, weight loss, appetite loss.

Risk Factors: High blood pressure, atherosclerosis.

ANGINA PECTORIS: Not a true disease, but a symptom of coronary atherosclerosis, which reduces blood supply of oxygen to the heart muscle.

Symptoms: Sharp pain around center of chest, often brought on by exercise or physical activity and eased by rest.

Risk Factors: Atherosclerosis, low blood sugar, too much insulin.

ARTERIOSCLEROSIS (Hardening of the Arteries): Loss of elasticity of arterial walls due to fatty plaque building.

Symptoms: Pain in calves of legs that is brought on by exercise and that disappears with rest. Pain in toes, severe at night and not eased by rest. May include dizziness, distortion of vision, stroke or heart attack.

Risk Factors: Same as **ATHEROSCLEROSIS**.

ATHEROSCLEROSIS: A disease of blood vessels involving fatty deposits called plaque building up on the insides of blood vessels.

Symptoms: None until disease is advanced, which may be indicated by leg cramps, angina pectoris, heart attack, stroke and other conditions.

Risk Factors: Stress, smoking, diabetes, high blood cholesterol, high blood pressure, kidney failure, alcohol abuse, lack of exercise, overweight, fatty diet, too much salt.

CARDIAC ARREST: Heart stops. May be caused by coronary artery disease or fibrillation in heart muscle.

Symptoms: Loss of consciousness. (Survival may depend on CPR application and calling ambulance or paramedics.)

Risk Factors: Same as atherosclerosis.

CARDIAC VALVE DISEASES: The four heart valves are subject to inflammation which causes thickening (stenosis) that prevents one or more valves from closing properly. Rheumatic fever and bacterial endocarditis (inflammation of the interior heart membrane) may cause valve diseases, which go by such names as mitral stenosis and incompetence, aortic stenosis and incompetence, tricuspid stenosis and incompetence and pulmonary stenosis and incompetence.

Symptoms: Breathlessness, weakness, fatigue.

Risk Factors: History of rheumatic fever or bacterial endocarditis.

CONSTRICTIVE PERICARDITIS: Inflammation of the outer heart membrane caused by a chronic infection. Long-term condition results in scarring or thickening or shrinking of the membrane so that heartbeat is impaired.

Symptoms: Swelling of legs and abdomen.

Risk Factors: Tuberculosis or other long-term infection.

CORONARY ARTERY DISEASE: (Coronary atherosclerosis, ischemic heart disease, coronary heart disease.)

Symptoms: Angina (pain around heart area), heart attack.

Risk Factors: Same as ATHEROSCLEROSIS.

CORONARY THROMBOSIS (Heart attack, myocardial infarction): Blockage of a coronary artery, resulting in cutoff blood supply and oxygen. Usually caused by a blood clot lodging in a coronary artery already partly blocked by atherosclerotic plaque.

Symptoms: A crushing pain in the center of the chest, or pain in the neck, jaw, arms and stomach. May be gradual, preceded by weeks of angina pain or may be sudden. Sensation can vary from tightness in chest to agonizing outburst of pain, either continuous, or a few minutes, or it may come and go for awhile. Symptoms may include nausea, light-headedness, sweating, dizziness, shortness or breath or fainting. There may be no symptoms at all in some cases, usually in the elderly.

Risk Factors: Same as ATHEROSCLEROSIS.

HEART FAILURE (and Congestive Heart Failure): Occurs due to loss of pumping ability by heart, due to muscle damage from disease or a valve defect. When the whole heart is affected, it is called **congestive heart failure**; when one side is affected, it is just **heart failure**. The name does not mean the heart has stopped working.

Symptoms: Left-Sided Heart Failure: Breathlessness, especially in the evening or after exercise. Difficulty breathing may become extreme. Lung congestion may produce bubbling sound. Also, maybe chest pain or blood-flecked sputum. **Right-Sided Heart Failure:** Fatigue, swelling of the ankles in those who can walk, swelling of lower back in the bedridden. Sometimes swelling of the liver. **Congestive Heart Failure:** Symptoms of left- and right-sided failure combined. Also loss of appetite and confusion.

Risk Factors: History of rheumatic fever, congenital heart defects.

HIGH BLOOD PRESSURE (Hypertension): High blood pressure is excessive pumping pressure of the blood by the heart. For a young person, blood pressure of 140/90 may be high. The upper figure represents the systolic pressure when the heart contracts to pump the blood. The lower pressure represents the pressure at relaxation between heartbeats. The numbers represent millimeters of mercury, a measurement of pressure. The cause of essential hypertension is unknown. The causes of secondary hypertension may be kidney disease, Cushing's disease, pregnancy or side effects of blood control pills.

Symptoms: None in early stages. Later stages, ringing in ears, headaches, general feeling of illness.

Risk Factors: Overweight, smoking, high salt intake. High blood pressure is twice as common in blacks as whites. People who have both high blood pressure and abnormal creatinine levels have a higher risk of death from heart attack or stroke than people who only have high blood pressure.

HYPERTROPHIC CARDIOMYOPATHY: Defective heart muscle cells, resulting in thickened heart walls.

Symptoms: Fatigue, chest pain, palpitations, shortness of breath.

Risk Factors: None known.

MYOCARDITIS: Inflammation of the heart muscle.

Symptoms: Shortness of breath and mild chest pain.

Risk Factors: None known.

NUTRITIONAL DEFICIENCY (**Cardiomyopathy**): Damage to the heart muscle due to vitamin or mineral deficiency or to effects of poison. Usually caused by deficiency of vitamin B-1 or potassium lack in blood.

Symptoms: Palpitations of heart, swollen hands and feet.

Risk Factors: Alcoholism, long-term use of diuretic drugs, chronic diarrhea.

PULMONARY EMBOLISM: Blood clot lodged in pulmonary artery, blocking blood flow in lung and reducing amount of oxygenated blood that returns to the heart.

Symptoms: Breathlessness, faintness, chest pain. Cough with bloody sputum. Blue around mouth. Rarely, collapse.
Risk Factors: Atherosclerosis.

VARICOSE VEINS: Twisted, swollen, disfigured veins, usually in legs, due to loss of valve efficiency. Varicose veins around anus are called hemorrhoids.
Symptoms: Appearance of bluish, enlarged, swollen, twisted veins.
Risk Factors: Pregnancy, work involving a lot of standing.

Recently, researchers have discovered a heart condition commonly mistaken in the past for a psychiatric disorder. Up to 100,000 women mostly in the middle-age range, in the U.S. may have this condition. According to the National Heart, Lung and Blood Institute, women who have had chest pains but no other signs of heart disease by the usual tests, have a disorder called "microvascular angina," blockage of the tiny arteries that nourish the heart. Doctors have previously mislabeled the condition as "neurotic" or "hysterical." Because these tiny arteries did not show up on angiograms, the problem remained hidden. We find that inadequate oxygenation and inadequate heart nutrition can also create heart problems that remain hidden for many years before they manifest with symptoms.

RHEUMATIC FEVER IN CHILDHOOD

Many children get rheumatic fever during their growing years. Rheumatic fever can be very mild or very severe, affecting some organs and parts of the body but not others. The heart is one of the organs sometimes affected. Damage to the heart valves may be permanent and very limiting to the person's lifestyle thereafter. Rheumatic fever is a streptococcal infection and may be so mild as to provide no noticeable symptoms at the time, but leaving serious after-effects, including possible heart damage.

INFLUENCES ON HEART FUNCTION

Many processes in our bodies can influence the way the heart works—and the level of its health.

These processes include nutrition, nerves, emotions, brain functions, glandular activities, gas in the stomach or bowel, digestion, assimilation, constipation, stress, exercise (or lack of it), attitudes, blood circulation, lymph circulation, oxygenation of the blood, obesity, drug side effects, alcohol intake, smoking, coffee, family life and relationships. Some persons are born with defective heart valves. Rheumatic heart disease can damage heart valves.

Where you live affects the risk level of heart disease and heart attack. The lowest death rates are in the Mountain, Pacific and West South Central regions of the U.S. The highest death rates are in the Middle Atlantic and East North Central regions. The difference may be in the relative amounts of natural calcium or sodium in the drinking water, or possibly the lack of minerals altogether. Lack of minerals or predominance of sodium could both increase heart attack risk.

A single source of aggravation to the heart—for example, a long-term potassium-deficient diet or constant high-stress life—can cause serious damage, but usually many factors are involved.

We will explore the many influences on heart function in this book and show what to do about each one.

Surely it was good advice which the Chinese gentleman gave to his American friend when he advised that in order to stay healthy, he should not overwork, he should get plenty of sleep, he should not get fat, and never, never get excited over anything.

THE GOOD NEWS FOR YOU

The good news about you and your heart is that by acting now, you may substantially change the lifestyle factors that are tearing down your heart, and you may greatly increase or improve those factors that build it up. This book may add years to your life if you properly apply what you learn from it, and may greatly improve the quality and level of enjoyment of the rest of your life.

With limited improvements in diet and exercise alone over the past few years, American men have reduced the number of deaths from cardiovascular disease by 25%. I feel that with the application of the ideas in this book, your cardiovascular system health will be raised to a level possibly unheard of in our time.

Good health is learned and earned—but you'll have to read this book before you begin earning health dividends.

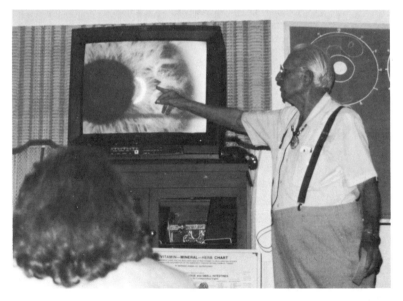

Dr. Jensen teaching an Iridology class of how degeneration shows up in the irides as black. He is pointing to the bowel area that is causing a reflex degenerate condition in the heart area. If you look at his Iridology chart, you will see that the degeneration is located over the heart area at 3 o'clock, in the left iris.

CHAPTER 4

THE CHOLESTEROL STORY

For some time now, the experts have been arguing over whether dietary cholesterol contributes to heart disease. The problem is, the body manufactures a good deal of cholesterol even when dietary cholesterol is kept very low, and there are some persons whose blood cholesterol remains abnormally high with a low food intake of cholesterol. So, in the past, researchers have had great difficulty agreeing on whether or not cholesterol in foods contributes to heart disease.

In October 1987, the Federal government and over 20 health organizations came out with detailed guidelines to the general public and physicians, stating that blood cholesterol levels should never be higher than 200 mg/dl, regardless of age or sex. Dietary guidelines called for a significant reduction in fat intake in our diets. The American Heart Association says that our daily diet should never be more than 30% fat. Some experts are saying our cholesterol should be under 180 mg/dl.

Cholesterol is a waxy substance found in foods such as milk, eggs, cheese and meat. It is also manufactured in the body by the liver. Cholesterol is a main ingredient of the artery-clogging plaque that signals arteriosclerosis, the primary cause of heart attack and stroke. Arteriosclerosis commonly goes with heart disease.

Plaque is a mix of cholesterol, fat, calcium and fibers that causes a progressive narrowing of arteries until the opening is so small that a blood clot can block it, leading to a heart attack or stroke.

TYPES OF CHOLESTEROL

There are different kinds of cholesterol, as follows:
VLDL: very low density lipoprotein cholesterol
LDL: low density lipoprotein cholesterol
HDL: high density lipoprotein cholesterol.
When we have our blood cholesterol tested, the number we see on the test report may be something like 212 mg/dl. This represents our **total** blood cholesterol, made up of all three kinds, measured in milligrams per deciliter.

Researchers are now calling LDL cholesterol "bad cholesterol" and HDL cholesterol "good cholesterol." They say we should cut down bad cholesterol and increase good cholesterol. Here is the reason why.

LDL cholesterol has been found to be one of the main fats deposited on the artery walls. The more LDL found in the blood, the greater the risk of heart disease. It is just the opposite with HDL.

HDL, or high density lipoprotein cholesterol, works to dissolve LDL from the plaque or artery walls. The higher the HDL level, the less risk of heart disease.

So, what is very low density lipoprotein (VLDL)?

Researchers say it is the substance used by the liver to make LDL, the bad cholesterol. The more VLDL cholesterol you have in your blood, the more LDL your liver can make.

Doctors talk about "the cholesterol ratio," meaning the ratio between the good cholesterol (HDL) and the bad cholesterol (LDL). When you have a blood test, it is a good idea to ask your doctor for the kind of cholesterol analysis that gives the HDL, LDL and VLDL results, as well as the HDL/LDL ratio.

Most blood tests give the level of triglycerides, a type of fat different from cholesterol. Researchers have found a connection between high cholesterol and high triglycerides. Lowering the triglycerides helps bring down the cholesterol level. Most Americans have levels of cholesterol and triglycerides that indicate an unnecessarily high risk of heart disease.

WHAT ABOUT OUR FOODS?

Research has shown that blood cholesterol levels between 140 and 180 mg/dl indicate the lowest risk of heart disease. When blood cholesterol rises above 200 mg/dl, the risk of heart disease increases significantly. So we need to adjust our food regimen and our level of regular exercise so that we bring our cholesterol level below the 200 mg/dl level.

There is a cautionary note to this cholesterol-lowering business that we are looking at. A 1989 study showed that there is a 600% increased risk of death from cerebral hemorrhage in those with cholesterol levels under 160 mg/dl who also have high blood pressure. Researchers speculate that very low blood cholesterol may be associated with weakened blood vessel walls that are more likely to break open if blood pressure gets too high. If the diastolic blood pressure is within normal limits, the risk disappears. The diastolic pressure is always the second (and usually lower) number on a blood pressure reading. If you have high blood pressure, it is best to set your blood cholesterol target no lower than 190 mg/dl.

How can we develop a safe low-blood cholesterol diet? My Health and Harmony Food Regimen fits the bill perfectly. I've been using this basic program for over 40 years (although not under the same name). The great advantage of my food regimen is that it strengthens the body and reduces the incidence of all disease, not just heart disease.

I advise throwing away the frying pan and avoiding all frying or cooking in hot oils. Cut out (or cut down) on the use of red meat. Increase the use of fish and poultry as protein sources. Avoid the use of concentrated oils for food purposes as much as possible. Increase your intake of fruits, vegetables and whole grains, having as much of your food raw as possible.

The "Healthy Heart Diet" of the American Heart Association recommends reducing the fat intake to 30% of the total calories. Animal fats (butter, cheese and fat on cooked meat) should be kept under 3% of the total calories in your diet. Get over 50% of your daily calories from vegetables, fruits and whole grains. Make your proteins about 15% of your daily calories. An artificial fat called "Simplesse" will be on the market by the time this book is published. I do not recommend any artificial foods.

Avoid organ meats, processed luncheon meats, bacon, sausage and foods cooked with lard, coconut or palm oil or shortening. Proctor and Gamble has an artificial fat for cooking now pending FDA approval. Avoid the artificial fats just as you avoid foods high in cholesterol. These are commendable improvements over dietary guidelines of past years.

WE NEED TO KNOW ABOUT LECITHIN

The problem with pointing out cholesterol as a "villain" (aside from the fact that there is such a thing as "good cholesterol—HDL") is the fact that our bodies need cholesterol. The very important point of safeguarding **dietary balance** between cholesterol and lecithin can be overlooked. Lecithin is a brain and nerve fat that is often found together with cholesterol in foods. It also makes up 80% of the male sexual fluid.

In foods in their natural, unprocessed state, lecithin balances cholesterol and keeps the cholesterol in a soluble form. We need both lecithin and cholesterol in every cell of our bodies and for coating nerves in the body and brain. The problem is that cooking destroys lecithin and leaves cholesterol intact. In my opinion, foods cooked at 212 degrees F. (the boiling point of water), retain their lecithin, while foods cooked at higher temperatures do not. When we use foods in which the lecithin is destroyed, only the cholesterol remains to circulate in the blood.

Eggs, which can be boiled or poached at 212 degrees F. are one of the finest proteins I know. The cholesterol is balanced by lecithin, and I do not believe that eggs cooked in the indicated manner will produce cholesterol that will deposit on the artery walls. However, fried or scrambled eggs, I believe, contribute to heart disease.

When lecithin is depleted in the body, cholesterol remains free to deposit on heart artery walls. If there is plenty of lecithin in the food, there is also plenty in the blood to keep cholesterol dissolved, to be used by the nerves and brain, and to replenish the sexual fluid. Excessive sex can deplete the body of lecithin, reducing the supply available for use by the rest of the body.

It is believed that lecithin is able to dissolve or remove cholesterol deposited on artery walls, but the evidence is not clear on this point. Nevertheless, because of the importance of lecithin in **preventing** cholesterol from depositing on heart artery walls, it is a very important nutrient in the prevention, control and, possibly, the reversal of heart disease. For that same reason, the sex drive should be kept under control in all kinds of heart trouble, because it can deplete lecithin by releasing too much of the sexual fluid.

An active sex life is important to overall health, but men with heart trouble will have to follow the rule of moderation in this regard. As we take care of the heart, using plenty of lecithin foods and being careful not to eat fried foods or foods cooked in oil, we also build up the nerves, brain and sexual system.

Lecithin is not only found in meat and eggs, but in raw nuts and seeds, including sesame seeds, so popular with the Turks. Sesame seed is a wonderful strengthening food for the heart and one of the finest lecithin foods. We will do well to make the lecithin foods an important part of our heart building regimen.

NIACIN AND CHOLESTEROL

In 1962, researchers reported that regular use of niacin (vitamin B-3) lowered cholesterol and triglycerides. In 1980, a study from Sweden reported that regular niacin intake reduced the risk of heart disease.

A University of Minnesota research report showed that taking niacin increased the good cholesterol while reducing the bad cholesterol.

Regular use of niacin in the Coronary Drug Project reduced the rate of non-fatal heart attack by as much as 21%.

One recent study has shown that for each 1% drop in blood cholesterol, the risk of having a heart attack drops by 2-3%. So a 10% reduction in cholesterol by using niacin would result in a lowering of a person's heart attack risk by 20-30%.

Because niacin causes a hot, tingling flush, bringing the blood to the face and upper extremities, experts recommend starting as low as 50 mg, three times per day, then increasing the dose every week until a whole gram is being taken three times daily. The niacin tablets should always be taken with food.

THE BRAN CRAZE

There is currently a bran craze going on that makes sense only because we have been using refined grains for so long, that we are bound to see wonderful benefits for a while from the taking of extra bran supplements. Taking supplementary bran is known to lower blood cholesterol.

I realize this is a heart book, but I can honestly say that we cannot have a healthy heart unless we have a healthy bowel—and a natural high-fiber diet is the best way to get it. We would not need to take bran supplements if we use sufficient amounts of fresh fruits, vegetables and whole grains in our daily food regimen.

In fact, Dr. James Cerda, a Florida doctor, was recently awarded the prestigious Paul Dudley White award for research showing how pectin-rich diets could help prevent atherosclerosis. He found out that grapefruit pectin lowered blood cholesterol, especially the "bad" cholesterol—LDL. In four months, volunteers taking 15 grams of grapefruit pectin daily lowered their cholesterol by 8%, even though they didn't change anything else in their diet. Pectin is considered a water-soluble fiber. Dr. Cerda recommends eating grapefruit, other citrus, carrots, Brussels sprouts, grapes and oat bran to reduce the risk of heart disease.

Another study called the "Lifestyle Heart Trial" showed that persons with blocked coronary arteries who could stick to a strict vegetarian diet, moderate daily exercise and stress reduction techniques could reverse the blockage, without cholesterol-lowering drugs. Those who made the biggest changes showed the best improvements. The 1990 study used 41 patients from San Francisco, ages 35 to 75 years. For exercise, the patients walked an hour a day. The late Nathan Pritikin was able to reverse arteriosclerosis for patients in his Santa Monica Clinic by an extreme low-fat diet together with a vigorous exercise regimen.

However, if you have been on a long-term diet of low-fiber foods and want to use fiber as a dietary supplement, here are my recommendations. I feel psyllium husks are probably the king of the fibers, although oat bran is currently the popular champion. Oat bran has both soluble and insoluble fiber, which reduces cholesterol both by removing it directly from the blood and by reducing bowel transit time. Some researchers believe that rice bran may be effective as oat bran in lowering cholesterol. Wheat bran, possibly the least expensive bran, primarily reduces bowel transit time.

STRESS REDUCTION

I want to mention one more interesting study. *The Journal of Human Stress* (**5**), 1979, carried an article by M.J. Cooper and M.M. Aygen titled "A Relaxation Technique in the Management of Hypercholesterolemia," showing that cholesterol levels could be lowered by relaxation techniques. This raises interesting questions.

Are blood cholesterol levels being increased by the stress of modern living in this country? Are we looking at a link between fast living and high cholesterol? Such questions can only be answered by future studies.

Finally, it is important for us to realize that cholesterol is a valuable nutrient, needed by every cell in the body. Our goal is simply to bring it into balance with respect to other nutrients in the diet.

What A Heartbeat Is Made Of

The heart almost becomes a secondary issue when we think of everything that has to be done properly for making the heart completely well. I think of the electrical impulses that trigger the heart beat, the oxygen required by the heart muscles, the nutrients, the blood that carries the oxygen and nutrients, the right blood pressure, the flexibility of arterial walls, the carrying off of metabolic wastes. There is so much to consider, so much to take care of.

CHAPTER 5

HIGH BLOOD PRESSURE

High blood pressure is exactly what the words indicate—excessive pressure against the walls of the arteries, like the pressure of air in a tire or the pressure of water in a water pipe. High blood pressure is also called hypertension and is considered a disease as well as a risk factor for arteriosclerosis, heart attack and stroke.

One of every six Americans has high blood pressure. Before I discuss high blood pressure, you should know what normal blood pressure is. Blood pressure is measured by an instrument called a sphygmomanometer (sfig-moh-ma-nom-i-tur). This consists of a hollow, inflatable cuff, a rubber bulb and tube used to pump air into the cuff, and a mercury pressure meter that looks like a big thermometer. When a nurse or doctor wraps a pneumatic cuff around your upper arm, pumps it up with the hand-squeezed rubber bulb, then listens through a stethoscope to the blood in your arm as pressure is released on the cuff, your blood pressure is measured.

The maximum pressure of the blood is when the heart contracts (systole) and thrusts the blood onward. This is called the systolic pressure. The lowest the blood pressure gets is between heartbeats (diastole) as the blood flows from one chamber of the heart to the other. This is the relaxation phase of the heart.

Normal blood pressure in a young man or woman would be about 120/70 where the 120 represents the systolic pressure, measured in millimeters of mercury, and the 70 represents the diastolic pressure. It is possible for the systolic pressure, in the case of high blood pressure, to get as high as 300, and for the diastolic pressure to get as high as 150. This would appear as a blood pressure reading of 300/150 on a blood pressure report. Blood pressure this high is dangerous.

There are two main kinds of high blood pressure. One kind includes all the sorts of high blood pressure where the cause is known. The other kind is called **essential hypertension** and it includes high blood pressure for which the cause is unknown. About 90% of high blood pressure cases are **essential hypertension.**

SYMPTOMS OF HIGH BLOOD PRESSURE

Some people have no symptoms when they are discovered to have high blood pressure in the doctor's office. Others report headaches, ringing in the ears (tinnitus), nosebleeds, insomnia or water retention in the tissues (edema). There may be a combination of symptoms.

Anyone who lives a high-stress lifestyle or has a high-stress job should have his blood pressure checked at least twice yearly.

The dilemma of the modern corporate executive is that the toll that stress exacts from his or her health is the price he or she often has to consider as a tradeoff for the excitement, challenge and financial rewards of work at that level of professionalism.

WHY IS HIGH BLOOD PRESSURE DANGEROUS?

High blood pressure is dangerous because it puts excessive strain on the heart and arteries and causes degenerative changes in their structure. Normally, the artery walls are flexible and can expand or contract to alter blood pressure as the body's needs change. High blood pressure can damage the arterial walls and cause hardening or even rupture.

Rupture of an artery of the brain can cause death or paralysis. This is called cerebral hemorrhage or stroke.

Scientific studies have shown that long-term high blood pressure increases the risk of heart disease (arteriosclerosis), stroke and kidney disease. Kidney disease, I should say, can also cause high blood pressure. These studies indicate that high blood pressure may create irritations or lesions that initiate hardening of the arteries (calcium and fat deposits). High blood pressure may also contribute to the plaque formation (fat deposits).

If we consider life insurance statistics, we find out that a 35-year-old man who has a blood pressure of, say, 150/100, is expected to have a life span 16 years shorter than he would if his blood pressure was 120/80.

Researchers have confirmed that the diastolic blood pressure is a reliable indicator of increased risk of death. An increase of 30 millimeters of mercury in the diastolic blood pressure doubles the risk of death. For example, the risk of death from brain hemorrhage increases six-fold in people with a blood cholesterol of 160 mg/dl or lower if they have a diastolic blood pressure reading over 90mm of mercury. This linkup of low cholesterol with high blood pressure apparently signals a weakening of the arterial walls that accounts for the increased strike risk.

BLOOD PRESSURE MEDICATIONS. ARE THEY SAFE?

People with high blood pressure are at a much greater risk of brain hemorrhage if they take aspirin or any other drug that hinders blood clotting. Aspirin has been recommended (one tablet every other day) to reduce the risk of a coronary heart attack. This procedure has proven itself very dangerous to those with high blood pressure.

No high blood pressure drugs are without side effects. Blood pressure drugs that dilate the blood vessels may cause water retention, heart palpitations or rapid heartbeat, or even drug-induced lupus (erythematosus). The kind that lowers blood pressure by increasing the urine output may deplete potassium, cause breast enlargement or increase uric acid and sugar in the bloodstream. Blood pressure pills classed as sympatholytics may have side effects such as impotence, depression, low energy, diarrhea or fever. I don't approve of using drugs for high blood pressure, excepting in extreme cases where no alternative therapy can be used.

RISK FACTORS IN HIGH BLOOD PRESSURE

In the United States, studies have shown that blood pressure increases with age, on the average. But, studies of people in other cultures show that blood pressure does not increase with age, necessarily. Research among the Yanomano Indians of Latin America shows that their average blood pressure actually goes down with age. During his studies of East African rural tribes, Dr. Denis Burkitt found almost no high blood pressure in rural natives of any age.

Black people in the U.S., on the other hand, have high blood pressure five times more frequently than the average white person, according to statistics from the U.S. Department of Health, Education and Welfare.

Aging, I believe, is not a risk factor or cause of high blood pressure. Instead, I believe that bad habits, over a long period of years, cause hardening of the arteries and changes in the heart and blood pressure, which contribute to high blood pressure. Most people in this country exercise too little, eat too much fatty food and become overweight. People here use too much salt and get too little calcium. These are the real villains in the hypertension story.

One interesting study showed that in people with a family history of high blood pressure, exposure to products containing the heavy metal cadmium can trigger the start of high blood pressure. Cadmium is found in cigarette smoke, industrial pollutants, seafood and even some drinking water supplies. Most people who have high blood pressure don't know how they got it and neither do their doctors, in most cases.

The Federal Trade Commission has charged that Campbell soups are not good for the heart, as Campbell's advertising has claimed, because some of the soups are high in sodium. A single serving of Campbell's chicken noodle soup, for example, contained 910 mg of sodium at the time they were tested.

Many risk factors have been considered as contributing to high blood pressure. Among them are hereditary stress, race, alcohol, overweight, smoking, salt, coffee and sedentary jobs. People with kidney disease often have high blood pressure. In fact, high levels of creatinine in the blood, often associated with the development or existence of kidney disease, have been shown to signal possible death from high blood pressure. Dr. Neil B. Shulman has stated, "More than 50% of people with a combination of high blood pressure and high levels of creatinine in the blood will die within eight years." Creatinine is a waste product of muscle metabolism which is usually filtered out of the blood by the kidneys.

APPROACHES TO REDUCING RISK FACTORS IN HIGH BLOOD PRESSURE

The recommendations I give for building a healthy heart will help bring down high blood pressure, but here are some other helpful tips.

If you are overweight, take off those extra pounds with the help of a good nutritional counselor or a nutrition-minded doctor. Then get on a no-weight gain food regimen such as My Health and Harmony Food Regimen and stay on it. Stop smoking and reduce or eliminate alcohol consumption. Exercise faithfully every day. Cut salt intake to under three grams a day. Throw out the coffee pot. Get rid of your frying pans.

Take sensible steps to reduce stress in your life (see my chapter on stress). Because stress depletes vitamins, especially B-Complex, it would be best to take a multi-vitamin supplement to make up for those deficiencies. Use more calcium-rich foods in the diet, and make sure you are getting some of the high-magnesium foods, since magnesium is needed for relaxation.

Calcium foods that I recommend include whole grains, seed and nut butters, yogurt, raw goat's milk, barley and kale soup and green vegetables. Avoid foods high in oxalic acid, which hinders absorption of calcium. These include spinach, chard, rhubarb, gooseberries, cranberries and chocolate.

High magnesium foods include yellow cornmeal, leafy green vegetables, chlorophyll, wheat germ, seed and nut butters, figs, soybeans and apples.

Using bread made of coarse-ground flour may help reduce high blood pressure. Digestion of fine flour bread can cause high blood insulin, which is suspected of being a cause of high blood pressure. Coarse-grain breads are also easier on the colon because of the higher fiber content. Keeping the colon clean and regular help control high blood pressure. Besides whole grains, potatoes, prunes and bananas are very high in fiber.

Nature walks are, in my opinion, wonderful for those with high blood pressure. The color green from the trees, shrubs and grass calms the mind. Deep breathing from a crisp-paced walk is recognized as helpful in lowering high blood pressure. The beauty of nature and the exercise combine to remove stress from the mind and body.

I don't like to bring religion into health matters, but we find that the spiritual life brings peace of mind to those who are sincere seekers of truth. My mother used to say, "If you lose your money, you have lost a lot, but if you lose your peace of mind, you have lost everything!" We need to keep peace of mind as one of our highest priorities in building a healthy cardiovascular system.

CHAPTER 6

DIET AND LIFESTYLE CHANGES

In the last 20 years, the U.S. death rate from heart disease has declined 40%. Doctors say the current death rate could be cut 50% more if people were willing to change their lifestyle factors that contribute to heart disease. Since the 1960s, the average diet dropped from 18% saturated fat to 13.5%. More adults are getting regular exercise, stopping smoking and lowering their blood pressure. High fiber foods are being used more. These are the factors lowering the cardiac death rate. High cholesterol and high fat diets are being blamed the most for heart disease.

Among environmental factors, "hard" drinking water high in calcium and magnesium may reduce the death rate due to heart attack or stroke by 10%. South Carolina, which has the highest level of soft water (high in sodium) in the country also has the highest stroke rate in the country. Cadmium in the drinking water, or in the polluted air of cities, triggers high blood pressure in those who have a family history of high blood pressure. Heart attacks are more likely to happen in the morning between 6 am and noon, while strokes are more likely in the Spring than at other times of the year. Fewer heart attacks and strokes take place in rural mountain areas such as the Caucasus mountains in Russia, Vilcabamba in Ecuador and the Hunza Valley in Pakistan. Simple low-fat diets and lots of walking are common factors in all three areas. The healthiest and most long-lived people I have ever met lived in those three parts of the world. Of course, diets higher in dairy products and meat are found to have the most cholesterol, and these are more available in Western nations.

Although cholesterol has been named as perhaps the main dietary villain in cardiovascular disease, we have to consider why cholesterol became such a problem in the past 50 years or so. Western nations were eating a great deal of red meat and dairy products (high cholesterol foods) long before the 20th century, so why wasn't heart attack common at that time? Studies of Eskimo tribes with high fat, high cholesterol diets have not shown any significant increase of cardiovascular disease. Considering these and other factors identified as contributing to cardiovascular disease, how can we make sense of what we know? And how can we do better?

WELCOME TO THE AGE OF TECHNOLOGY

When we think of automobiles, stereos, jet planes, computers and other symbols of our high-tech age, it seems that man is making substantial progress in civilization. But, when we look at disease statistics, we wonder where we've gone wrong. There's a good side to technology and progress, and a bad side as well. Sometimes we don't realize the changes created in our lives by the impact of technology.

Smoking of tobacco, for example, was introduced by the American Indians to the early European explorers and settlers, but cigarette manufacture and extensive "social smoking" didn't really begin in earnest until the 1930s. Even as late as the 1950s, smoking by women was still frowned upon, while cigarette smoking has become an addictive practice with millions of men and a smaller, but significant, population of women.

It would seem that tobacco smoking did not become widespread until 20th century manufacturing, distributing and advertising processes created the illusion that smoking cigarettes, cigars, pipes and so forth makes a person appear more sophisticated, intelligent, socially acceptable, physically attractive and sexually desirable. The successful marketing of an addictive drug like tobacco to millions of Americans reveals one of the most undesirable aspects of modern technology.

Likewise, the food processing industry developed, manufactured, promoted and distributed thousands of refined, packaged and chemically "treated" foods and food products that were not available prior to the 20th century. Mass manufacturing kept the prices low to make products attractive to consumers, but the health impact of so much devitalized, chemically processed food on nations accustomed to a more wholesome, down-to-earth diet carries all the earmarks of disaster.

The widespread manufacture of cars in the 20th century, together with innumerable "labor saving" devices for home and work place, and entertainment like films, television and spectator sports have made legs almost obsolete and rear ends indispensable. People in this country do more sitting than almost anything else, and this has weakened the heart muscles of millions of persons who suffer from a chronic lack of exercise.

Life in the 1800s as compared to life in the 1900s was slower-paced, characterized by a greater emphasis on "thinking things over" before acting, taking life one step at a time, emphasizing quality over quantity and appreciation of individuality. It was not uncommon in the 1800s for young men and women to be engaged from 2-to-5 years before getting married. In contrast, the 20th century could be called the Age of Stress, Speed and Noise—freeways, jet airports, computers, instant everything. Everyone wants everything done yesterday, if not sooner. This is distinctly a 20th century contribution to the deterioration of health in modern cultures, as shown in Hans Selyes' classic book, *The Stress of Life*.

Medicinal drugs as well as illicit addictive drugs like heroin, cocaine, methamphetamines and others became widespread in this century. They were available to a far less extent in the last century. Many drugs are actually or potentially harmful to the heart, alone or in combination with other drugs, food chemicals and dangerously imbalanced diets. Even heart drugs can be dangerous to the heart. Drugs used to treat irregular heartbeat, like procainamide, tocainide and encainide were found to make many patients worse, and even increased risk of death. Alcohol abuse, which is widespread, should be included in the category of drugs dangerous to the heart.

Homogenized milk which is produced by forcing pasteurized milk at high pressure through a fine screen, has been implicated as a possible contributing factor in arteriosclerosis. Some researchers assert that an enzyme harmful to the artery walls becomes "trapped" in fat particles during homogenization, and is absorbed through the bowel wall and into the bloodstream, where it attacks the linings of cells that make up arterial walls.

The 20th century has produced a working class and middle class of the U.S. that can afford dairy products and beef associated with high cholesterol, high heart-risk diets. Surprisingly, the heart disease rate decreases as wealth increases, according to researchers. The rich seem to have changed the lifestyle factors that lead to heart disease, while the workers and white color people lag far behind. By and large, however, modern life is hard on the heart.

Do you get the picture? Can you see how cultural change can create a whole new "lifestyle," with many new and different products and processes that affect our health in revolutionary ways?

Nevertheless, we can take steps to improve our personal heart health, once we know what dietary and lifestyle changes are dangerous to our health and what to substitute in their place.

LET'S GET SPECIFIC

As I have said in an earlier chapter, "The Cholesterol Story," the first step in reducing cardiovascular risk should be to throw out the frying pan. The fatty deposits on arterial walls are mostly made of saturated or "animal" fat and cholesterol. While some saturated fat and some cholesterol is needed for a healthy body, most of us use too much. A Western Electric

Company study of 1,900 male employees, aged 40-45, for 20 years found that those who ate more fat had over 1/3 more heart attacks than those who ate less fat. We shouldn't be eating foods soaked in fat at all! The American Heart Association recommends limiting our daily fat intake to 30% of our total dietary calories. Keep your total blood cholesterol under 200 md/dl and try to keep your high density lipoprotein (good cholesterol) over 40 mg/dl. Watching fat intake is an important step, but you also need sufficient exercise and vitamin supplements to bring your fat and cholesterol blood levels to a safe place. A person with a blood cholesterol level of 300 mg/dl has four times the chance of getting a heart attack as a person with a blood cholesterol of 200 mg/dl.

A recent government report showed that the average American's blood cholesterol would be lowered 10% and nationwide heart disease would be lowered 20% if people ate less fat—no more than 30% of dietary calories per day.

RED MEAT AND SALT

Reduce red meat (pork and beef) to once or twice a week and lower salt intake as much as you can. If you are a heavy salt user, try substituting the vegetable/herbal seasonings available at your local health food store. You may like one better than others, so experiment. No one is sure why red meat increases the risk of heart disease (besides its fat content) but statistics show it does, so cut down. Table salt, which is sodium chloride, may contribute to high blood pressure and cardiovascular disease by interfering with the sodium/potassium balance in the body. It would be best to eliminate it from your diet but if you must have it, use as little as possible and rely more on other seasonings.

Refined Sugar. Studies show that a high sugar intake is associated with elevated blood cholesterol. In a recent study, the average person in the U.S. was found to have an annual sugar intake of 130 pounds, **five times the sugar intake of the turn**

of the century. Diabetes, a widespread sugar metabolism disorder, is associated with a high incidence of heart disease, at an earlier age than normal.

Lack of Exercise. Exercise moves the venous blood back to the heart and increases the oxygenation level of the blood. Exercise is necessary to keep the circulatory system moving well, to burn up excess calories and to strengthen the heart muscle. "Use it or lose it," the saying goes. Most Americans get far too little exercise, which contributes to weakening the heart and lowering the oxygen intake.

Smoking Cigarettes. Smokers have double the heart attack risk of nonsmokers. Men and women who smoke 25 or more cigarettes each day may have 10-to-15 times the risk of heart disease as nonsmokers.

Obesity. Obesity increases the load on the heart by simply providing extra pounds for the body to carry around and hundreds of miles more fine blood vessels running through the extra fatty tissue. It also increases the chance of getting diabetes, which increases heart disease risk. Avoid fad diets. Ask your doctor to recommend a weight-loss diet for you or read my book *Slender Me Naturally*.

Stress. A survey for the American Academy of Family Physicians some years ago covered six occupational groups and found that the job site was the greatest single producer of stress leading to adverse health. A more recent study says that conflicts with people on the job, family members and other associates is the primary source of stress for the average person. Both are likely to be sources of high stress, along with such events and processes as freeway driving, divorce, death of a loved one, financial problems and exposure to high levels of noise. Men hold anger longer than women do, and tend to be less effective in dealing with stress.

Alcohol Use and Abuse. Analysis of 1,968 men and 2,505 women in the Framingham Heart Study showed that heart disease risk increased with even a drink of two a day for middle-aged men. Use of alcohol is linked with oversized heart and the development of abnormal heartbeats, forcing the heart to pump harder. The risk increases with age, overweight, high blood pressure and number of drinks per day. Women have a lower risk than men. Previous studies had shown that alcohol was toxic to heart tissue, and that persons who had three or more drinks per day had higher blood pressure than those who drank less. A Gallup poll showed that 69% of adult Americans drink, while 9% 18 and 29 years old, 80% drink. The evidence is growing to favor the idea that it is better not to drink alcoholic beverages at all.

High Blood Pressure. A major cardiovascular research project, the Framingham Study, showed that for every 10mm increase in blood pressure there was a 30% increased risk of stroke. You should see your doctor if you have high blood pressure and do what you need to do to bring it down.

Sources of Heart Strain. Any sudden shock or excessive or prolonged stress on the cardiovascular system can cause heart strain on a heart unaccustomed to such burdens or on a congenitally weak heart. We must be careful of such things as: Sudden strenuous movements, cold water bathing, wrestling, boxing, fighting; exposure to cold, wind and drafts; athletic performance/games; exposure to excessive heat; running or climbing; crowds and crowded halls, where air is close and stale; heavy lifting; running up stairs; exposure to smoke, chemical fumes, gases; heavy meals; late hours; ice-cold drinks; overwork; vigorous physical dancing; worry, depression or fear; gymnastic workout; unaccustomed exposure to high altitudes; stormy arguments; bodily chill or overheating; and loud, sudden noises.

If you know you are going to be facing situations involving difficult, heavy exertion in the future, spend time in workouts to build your body, heart and lungs before you get there. Overexertion with an out-of-shape body is asking for trouble, perhaps heart trouble.

A HEART-TO-HEART TALK

We must be willing to stop doing what is breaking our bodies down before we start building our bodies up. I have been working in nutrition for over 60 years, and I can tell you this: You can break your body down faster than any health regimen can build it back up.

If you really want a healthy heart and circulatory system, you must commit yourself, first, to stop those lifestyle habits and factors that are actually or potentially harming your heart. So many smokers and heavy alcohol users have waited until they had their first heart attack to stop drinking and smoking. They generally stopped because their doctor would say, after the heart attack,"If you don't quit, you're going to die." Now that is very harsh, I realize, but very true.

In a later chapter, we will discuss a strategy for successfully making lifestyle changes, but in this chapter, I simply want to point out how lifestyle events and processes may combine, interact and accumulate to tear down your heart and pave the way for a heart attack or stroke unless you do something about it.

What the Heart Needs Most
or "If You Love Your Heart, Take Care of It!"

My work has been in the wholistic health field which takes into account nutrition, exercise, attitude, constitutional weakness, effects of stress and the sum total of contributions of body and mind to any particular health problem. I feel it is of the utmost importance to point out that in taking care of the heart, we must do everything possible to increase the supportive activity of the rest of the body. If we're going to properly care for the heart that God gave us, we have to make sure that the whole family of organs is working as one. All organs, glands and tissues must be brought to the best possible level of function for the heart to respond well to surgical intervention or other procedures.

CHAPTER 7

STRESS AND YOUR HEART

On a quiet morning in May, 1991, President Bush was jogging at Camp David, Maryland, when his heart rate began to increase and became irregular. He sensed the irregular heartbeat, became short of breath and was taken immediately to a doctor. What caused this heart fibrillation? Let's look at what the President's week had been like.

Iraq's Saddam Hussein scoffed at President Bush's desire to oust him. Vice President Quayle and Chief of Staff John Sununo were accused of squandering taxpayers' money in the press and on TV. A U.S. move to restore Mid-East peace was rejected. The President knocked himself out lifting weights, playing tennis, shooting baskets and doing aerobics to kick off National Fitness and Sports Month. He was accused of dealing with the Iranians to manipulate an election issue in 1980. He flew to and from St. Louis on Friday, flew Saturday to and from the University of Michigan to give a speech before the graduating class, then left for Camp David to relax, rest and take an easy jog. Is it any wonder his heart began to react to all that stress?

Because our heart, lungs, blood pressure and circulation are directly influenced by the "chest brain" in the medulla oblongata, and indirectly influenced by other parts of the brain and by the endocrine system, the health of our cardiovascular system is intimately related to how well we handle our emotional responses to the events we encounter in life.

When you are under stress, your blood pressure increases, blood vessels constrict and your heart pounds. Stress is hard on the heart and arteries.

We live in fast times. Over 20 million Americans suffer from anxiety disorders. There have been more changes in the 20 century than all the rest of history altogether. Our particular era has been dubbed, variously, the industrial age, the technical age, the space age, the computer age, the information age, the jet age, the electronic age—names that imply speed, rapid change, challenge.

When I was a young boy, hearing music from a radio seemed almost a miracle. I remember looking up into the sky at airplanes, wondering what on earth could keep them in the air. Now we have put men on the moon, and we communicate around the world instantly by orbiting satellite relay stations.

Change causes stress. The rule is, the more change, the more stress. If we fight or resist change, we suffer adverse consequences from stress far more than if we learn to live with change, accept change, make our peace with change. Young people used to say, "You have to go with the flow." It's true. For the sake of our own health and peace of mind, we have to learn to "go with the flow."

Stress is a word that is relatively new in its application to health, but it is one of the most dangerous risk factors yet discovered in research on heart disease. Stress is dangerous because it is invisible, because it can creep up on an unsuspecting person without warning.

THE SOLDIER'S HEART

My friend and teacher, V.G. Rocine, coined an expression for wartime stress that he called "the soldier's heart." Soldiers in wars are compelled to bear hardships of every variety. They are exposed to rain, sleet, hail, snow, heat, exhaustion, danger, sleeplessness and overwork, at the very least. This all affects the soldier's heart.

The soldier's nutrition in wartime is none the best, especially with bullets flying overhead and shells or bombs bursting nearby. Stress and adrenaline interfere with digestion, and excessive fear acids are secreted and carried by the blood and lymph. Canned foods loaded with preservatives are eaten in the trenches. There may be no fresh fruit or vegetables for weeks at a time. This is hard on the whole body, especially the soldier's heart.

The battlefront may be a place where close friends are lost in a moment, where the cries of the wounded are heard over the din of battle. Extreme fear causes a feeling of suffocation. Nerves are on edge, and tempers flair. Hands sweat and shake, and the heart trembles.

Without proper food, exposed to extremes of physical and mental stress, the soldier's heart can be severely damaged. But, even in peacetime, stress takes a great toll on people.

WE LIVE IN AN AGE OF STRESS

The importance of stress is undeniable. Its purpose in life is to aid survival and stimulate us to higher levels of performance. The problem is, stress can be destructive inside us if we don't handle it properly. Stress is pressure, caused by our reaction to disturbing situations. Stress enters our lives when we are alarmed, upset or challenged.

We are all familiar with stories about persons who die of heart attacks after hearing that their business has suddenly become bankrupt, or their child has been killed in an auto accident. We recognize that the cause of such heart attacks is not the gradual progress of heart disease to a stage of crisis, but the shock of bad news. This shock is part of the stress response.

Stress can also build up more slowly. Workaholics are notorious for heart attacks and strokes in their middle-to-late years. It is not difficult to see how the accumulated pressure of a daily 12-to-15 hour grind, week after week, year after year, could end up in a disease crisis, resulting in a heart attack. Men and women in demanding jobs with little freedom to make decisions have three times the risk of getting high blood pressure than people in less stressful jobs.

PHYSICAL PRESSURE

Any pressure brought on the heart and continued for a while affects the heart and its workings. Overweight people who try to sleep on their stomachs may find that pressure is brought against the heart. Likewise, gas due to indigestion may bring pressure against the heart, as well as the liver, spleen, pancreas and so on. This, too, is stress. Whether the pressure source is external or internal, the heart is under stress and its performance is hindered, if only a little.

Cooked squash can reduce gas in the digestive tract. Sulfur foods should be avoided. Herbal teas such as fenugreek and peppermint, help get rid of gas. A cup of boiling water plus a tablespoon of Capri Mineral Whey (dried goat whey), four drops of oil of peppermint and a teaspoon of liquid chlorophyll is sometimes a great help with gas.

RUNNER'S HEART OR ATHLETE'S HEART

A problem just as shocking, sudden and surprising as infant crib death is "runner's" or "athlete's" heart, in which can athlete in his prime dies suddenly during exercise. What is surprising is that long distance running is known to strengthen the heart and slow the pulse, yet long distance runners have died suddenly of heart attacks.

RESEARCH ON STRESS

Stress was studied in great detail and depth in the 1940s and 1950s by a scientist named Hans Selye. Dr. Selye learned about stress by studying the body's reactions to many different kinds of injury, diseases, poison, over-stimulation or unusual workload. He found that temperature extremes, smoke, noise, arguments, grief, joy—and even vacations—could cause stress that resulted in internal chemical and physical changes in the body.

Dr. Selye defined stress as "nonspecific response of the body to any demand made on it," whether the situation creating the demand is a good experience or a bad experience. Notice that stress is not defined by what happens "outside us" but by what happens "inside us."

Our response to stress, the internal changes that take place, are called the **general adaptation syndrome**. When we come under stress, research has shown that three things happen.

First, we experience an **alarm stage**. Our minds and/or bodies encounter the stress-producing situation—whether it is a burn, loss of a job, the wedding of an adult child, an earthquake or divorce makes no difference. The alarm stage triggers certain body responses.

The second stage is the **resistance stage**, where the body begins to adapt to the continuing consciousness of whatever is causing the stress. The adrenal glands release the hormone adrenaline, which almost immediately raises the blood pressure, increases the heart rate, increases the blood sugar level, dilates the bronchial tubes and prepares the body for emergency action. Hormones from the thyroid and the pancreas are also released during the **resistance stage**.

When the period of stress is prolonged, the **stage of exhaustion** is reached. It is during this stage that disease can be initiated in inherently weak organs, glands and tissues of the body. Over many months or even years, the effects of stress, particularly exhaustion, lower the level of immune system function so a person can no longer resist a disease. The adrenal and thymus glands become depleted, the lymph nodes are less active, and the stomach lining becomes irritated.

Stress-related diseases and afflictions include stomach ulcers, high blood pressure, colitis, atherosclerosis, asthma, arthritis, skin problems, irritable bowel syndrome, heart attack and stroke.

As a person encounters a stressful event, the feelings he or she has triggers responses in the brain, nervous system and endocrine system. Over-stressed persons, or chronically-stressed persons, overstimulate glands and organs in their bodies—particularly the heart. This kind of reaction invites disease. Lowered immunity due to stress is possibly why many people come down with a cold or flu, even though they have been living with the virus that brings on the condition without getting sick.

With the onset of stress, the development of the **resistance stage** to that particular source of stress causes a lowering of resistance to other pre-existing sources of stress, such as chronic disease. According to researchers, that is why many elderly persons with existing chronic diseases die when a flu epidemic comes along.

Worry is a type of low-level stress. When Dr. V.G. Rocine was asked to comment on the effects of worry on the heart, he had this to say: "Disappointment in love, worry about children, grief over loved ones and the breakup of a love relationship eat at the heart, dry up the secretions, depress the circulation, darken the mind and ruin the health." In other words, worry can contribute to heart trouble.

THE FIGHT OR FLIGHT SYNDROME

We should realize that not everyone responds the same way to a stressful situation. When the sales manager of a company tells his salesmen, "I'm giving all of you responsibility for increasing sales by 15% next month," some of the salesmen relish the challenge, while others view it with fear and dread.

Spotting a rattlesnake beside a hiking path will have an entirely different impact on a biology teacher and on a bank clerk who is afraid of snakes.

When our minds interpret a situation as threatening, the autonomic nervous system of the brain triggers a stress response more commonly known as the "fight or flight" syndrome. The body's reaction is very much like that described in the **resistance stage of stress**: increased blood pressure and heart rate, release of blood sugar, bronchials dilate to get more oxygen into the lungs, dilation of pupils and increased alertness of the brain.

We are prepared to fight or run away, whichever is necessary, possible or wiser (provided we have a choice). In more primitive conditions than our current culture, the act of fighting or running would "use up" the energy and adrenaline secreted. When we can't fight or run, as in the case of an employer exploding with anger when an employee has made a mistake, the internalized or bottled up "fight or flight" response is very destructive. Cases have been recorded, for example, where men have had heart attacks due to fear and surprise generated from watching movies or television. Films like "Jaws" which picture a giant shark attacking a swimmer or small boat, can cause the "fight or flight" syndrome right inside the safety of a movie theater. Movies or TV programs intended to generate horror, fear or shock should be avoided by all who have cardiovascular problems.

Once upon a time, the "fight or flight" syndrome was caused by real tigers, marauding pirates and news of an approaching cholera epidemic. Now it is caused, vicariously, by soap operas, by shock and horror films, by wars, atrocities, accidents and crimes on TV news. The "fight or flight" syndrome is also encountered in modern urban life but in new forms.

Violent crimes like mugging, assault, rape and murder are more common than ever. Attacks on women and the elderly are more frequent than any other period in history. Auto accidents triggered by drunk or drugged drivers make freeway driving a risky gamble with one's life and divorce and unhappy marriages are common. Air pollution stresses the lungs. Noise pollution stresses the brain.

Economic ups and downs, stock market tumbles, employment layoffs, industrial mergers resulting in massive reorganizations, taxes, foreign investment or ownership of local businesses, rising prices, the shocking expense of modern health care—these and other events of our time can be just as jolting, shocking, enraging, tragic and stressful as tribal warfare in a primitive culture.

WARNING SIGNS OF STRESS

Some of the warning signs that stress is reaching serious levels in your life are accident proneness, nervousness, irregular heartbeat, sleeplessness, irritability, difficulty in concentrating and loss of muscle coordination. Sieges of anxiety with sweating palms of the hands and sweating eyelids are sometimes experienced. Even though you may realize that "flight" is impossible, you may fantasize often on escaping from your troubles, getting away to some Shangri-la. Unexplainable nausea, vomiting or diarrhea may be signs of stress buildup. If you aren't sure, check with your doctor. Most doctors these days can recognize stress symptoms and tell the difference between stress consequences and illness.

STRATEGIES FOR DEALING WITH STRESS

When you know there is nowhere to escape and that you can't fight changes that are part of our time, part of our culture, the only other thing you can do is try to keep your peace of mind and make your home into a pleasant, relaxing refuge from the storm. Use calm, pleasant colors in your home—soft, relaxing colors like white, cream, pastels like yellow, pink and blue. Put up cheerful wallpaper and pleasant decorations. Make your home into a "wellness center," as I have often advised.

Watch only uplifting programs on TV. Play soft and soothing music on the stereo. Take naps when possible.

Exercise is a wonderful antidote to stress, but if you have cardiovascular disease, don't try to exercise without consulting your doctor. We have an entire chapter on exercise in this book.

Actively work to build up your own health and to keep a cheerful, positive frame of mind. Cultivate active, warm friendships and healthy, loving relationships within your family. Show your affection by touching those you love. Expressions of love such as hugs and kisses are health building. Stay away from bitter, spiteful people. Avoid unnecessary arguments and disagreements.

I have heard that the Chinese word for "crisis" is made up of the symbols for danger and opportunity. Look for the bright side in every unexpected or discomforting experience you encounter. Look for the opportunity to learn something new, to do something for yourself or others in the circumstances.

When you anticipate and accept stressful events and situations as a normal part of your future and plan in advance to respond to them as courageously and gracefully as you can, the fear and dread so often associated with the unknown and unexpected goes away.

Those who follow a spiritual path and make religion an important part of their life often seem to keep afloat when others are sinking.

Make sure you are using a balanced diet to prevent stress damage. Certain vitamins and minerals are believed to help fight stress. These include vitamins B-Complex, C and E and minerals such as zinc, calcium, magnesium and potassium. Try to get most of your vitamins and minerals from food. If you are over 50, it is reasonable to take a multi-vitamin and mineral tablet with meals.

Avoid foods and drinks that increase or aggravate stress. Cut down on salt and cut out refined sugar, fried foods, fatty meats, tea, coffee, cola drinks, chocolate and junk foods of all kinds.

Stress creates harmful, undesirable acids in the body. Eating refined carbohydrates such as sugar, white flour, white rice and products made from them (cakes, pies, etc.) increases body acids and depletes sodium, potassium, magnesium and calcium from the body. (These are acid-neutralizing chemical elements, and it is best to get them in foods rather than supplements.) An overall acidic condition in a body depleted of acid-neutralizing salts creates a favorable environment for illness and disease—a fatigued body with irritated nerves, poor digestion and a suppressed immune system.

The first thing an over-stressed person needs to do is to identify lifestyle events and choices that are tearing down his health and eliminate them. I mean things like staying out too late (or staying up too late), always rushing to get somewhere on time, alcohol abuse, smoking, overeating, lack of exercise, chronic complaining, chronic debts and poor money management, drug abuse, a critical attitude and lack of exercise. You have to stop breaking down before you can build yourself up. This is especially important when you are over-stressed.

The next thing is to start a recovery and rebuilding program, focussing on improved physical well-being and getting your mental attitude in shape.

WHAT IS YOUR LIFE CHANGE TEST SCORE?

Go over the following list of common sources of stress in everyday life and find your total life change score by adding up the points assigned to events on the list that have happened to you in the past year. If you score below 150 points, you need not expect health problems due to stress. If you score over 300 points, you will need to get to work on an effective health-building program. The test was developed by Drs. T.H. Holmes and R.H. Rahe.

STRESS RATING SCALE

Rank	Life Event	Stress Rating
1	Death of spouse	100
2	Divorce	73
3	Marital separation	65
4	Jail term	63
5	Death of close family member	63
6	Personal injury or illness	53
7	Marriage	50
8	Fired from job	47
9	Marital reconciliation	45
10	Retirement	45
11	Change in health of family member	44
12	Pregnancy	40
13	Sex difficulties	39
14	Gain of new family member	39
15	Business readjustment	39
16	Change in financial state	38
17	Death of a close friend	37
18	Change to different line of work	36
19	Change in number of arguments with spouse	35
20	Mortgage over $10,000	31
21	Foreclosure of mortgage or loan	30
22	Change in responsibilities at work	29
23	Son or daughter leaving home	29
24	Trouble with in-laws	29
25	Outstanding personal achievement	28
26	Wife begins or stops work	26
27	Begin or end school	26
28	Change in living conditions	25
29	Revision of personal habits	24
30	Trouble with boss	23
31	Change in work hours or conditions	20
32	Change in residence	20
33	Change in schools	20
34	Change in recreation	19
35	Change in church activities	19
36	Change in social activities	18
37	Mortgage or loan less than $10,000	17
38	Change in sleeping habits	16
39	Change in number of family get-togethers	15
40	Change in eating habits	15
41	Vacation	13
42	Christmas	12
43	Minor violations of the law	11

Stress, like life itself, is full of the predictable and the unexpected, as is demonstrated by this list ranking 42 common experiences in terms of stress.

TEN STEPS TO QUICK STRESS RELIEF

1. Don't hold resentments or feelings of being unfairly treated. Talk it over as soon as possible with the person you have negative feelings about.

2. Learn to control your anger (not bottle it up) by deciding not to get mad when you are in a conflict situation. If your boss attacks you, say, "Let's calm down and take care of this problem."

3. Take 10 deep breaths, holding each breath for a count of 15 and exhale slowly.

4. Pray, by talking to God as you would another person, sharing your feelings (including anger or resentment) about the person or situation causing the stress.

5. Forgive and forget if someone has wronged you. Just say to yourself, "I forgive (him/her) for doing such-and-such." Being unforgiving is a source of stress.

6. Let the tears come. Whether you are a man or a woman, crying is one of the best ways to release frustration, grief or anger.

7. Take a walk—for about half an hour. Walking reduces nerve and muscle tension, helping you to relax.

8. Take a long, warm soak in the bathtub. Close your eyes and relax.

9. Do something you enjoy—take in a movie, go to a museum, drive up to the mountains, take a nature hike, phone someone you love.

10. Go somewhere with a friend and talk your situation over. Talking things over often puts in a more realistic perspective, making you feel better about your situation.

CHAPTER 8

CIRCULATION IS LIFE

The Good Book says, "The life of the body is the blood," and we find that either blockage of an artery, as in heart attack, or the bursting of a blood vessel, as in stroke, can bring a sudden end to life. Circulation of the blood is the primary purpose of the heart, for the circulation of the blood is vital to the life of all parts of the body.

Nature is our true friend. Good, clean blood is our best medicine and a correct diet our only salvation in a case of heart disease.

At any given time, 20% of the entire oxygen supply of the bloodstream is being used in the brain to feed and energize the nerve system. Another large percentage of the oxygen is used by the heart. Any interruption of the oxygen supply to the brain or heart for even a few minutes results in severe tissue damage. Brain damage always affects the body. Heart damage affects the brain.

Taber's Encyclopedic Medical Dictionary refers to the blood as an "organ," and it must be classified as a vital organ, for when it stops moving, life stops.

For this reason—that is, the importance of blood—I have studied the circulatory system very carefully. While the heart is the pump that circulates the incoming venous blood through the lungs and the outgoing arterial blood to the organs and body tissues, it is the legs that pump the venous blood back to the heart.

WHEN BLOOD CIRCULATION
BECOMES INADEQUATE

It isn't growing older that slows and hinders the circulation of the blood, it is inactivity, poor nutrition and laziness. Fatigue and the wasting of vitality due to poor health habits bring on increasing inactivity, and this, in turn, leads to slowed circulation. With slower circulation less oxygen is carried to the brain and heart, which reduces their level of function. Unless a determined act of the willpower changes the situation, the result is a downward spiral in health—especially cardiovascular health.

When blood circulation becomes inadequate, all tissues of the body are inadequately fed and oxygenated, but the brain is affected the most. This is very serious, because the brain regulates metabolism, the endocrine system and the level of every function of every organ and tissue of the body. When brain functions slow the whole body becomes sluggish and underactive.

Poor circulation, if not corrected, soon becomes poor health. If the circulation of the blood is poor, circulation of the lymphatic system (which relies on muscular activity) is also poor. The lymphatic system is the heart of our natural immune system, and its breakdown is an invitation to disease. Fatigue and low vitality are the first symptoms.

BRINGING CIRCULATION ACTIVITY BACK

Nutrition and exercise are the twin keys for reversing fatigue, low vitality and blood circulation. Let's look at nutrition first.

The heart, being primarily a muscle, gets its main chemical need of potassium from food. But because the heart is also composed of membranes, tendons and ligaments, it needs a certain amount of sodium also. We don't want the sodium from table salt, which behaves more like a drug than a food in the body, but we need food sodium. And to meet the other chemical needs of the heart and vascular cells, we need calcium, silicon, lecithin, and, of all things, a little cholesterol. In the following chapter, I will discuss feeding the heart more specifically, but here the main thing to realize is that the heart, having been deprived of nutrients, needs to have them restored.

Think about what that means. For the heart to get the nutrition it requires, we have to make sure the digestion is good, which means that the stomach, small intestines, liver, gallbladder and pancreas must all be working efficiently and in harmony. Also as nutrients come in, wastes must be carried out, so we have to make sure the kidneys, skin, lungs and bowel are all eliminating properly. We have to have friendly flora in the bowel, so we may use a little acidophilus culture as a dietary supplement.

We can't just feed the heart. We must also feed every organ, gland and tissue that supports the heart or interacts with the heart. So, we feed the whole body, adding supplements that will speed up and enhance the restoration of chemical balance in the body. We will, of course, need iron-rich foods to build the blood, allowing more oxygen to be carried to the tissues.

Our nutritional support program must be accompanied by exercise and other means of stimulating circulation.

HOW CAN WE STIMULATE CIRCULATION?

Walking is the best all around exercise for the heart and circulation. Dr. Paul Dudley White, a prominent heart specialist who treated President Dwight D. Eisenhower, used to say, "The legs are the pumps that drive the venous blood back to the heart." Walking not only drives the circulation, but increases the metabolic rate. This, in turn, raises the activity level of every organ, gland and tissue in the body, allowing them to assimilate nutrients faster and get rid of wastes more speedily. All forms of manipulation: massage, chiropractic, osteopathy, acupuncture, Shiatsu and others will assist in restoring circulation and making sure nerve supply is open and working well.

There's no use trying to improve heart health, function and strength when other organs and body systems are dragging it down by their own low level of function.

We can take vitamin E to increase oxygenation but we also may need to take up breathing exercises.

Barefoot walks in the early morning in sand or grass (both, if possible) are wonderful stimulants to the circulation.

I have visited the Kneipp baths at Worishofen, Germany, where people waded through channels of cold water, then let their legs dry by evaporation in the sunshine. Father Sebastian Kneipp believed that cold water was "live" water and advocated the use of cold water baths to stir up the circulation. Kneipp baths can be simulated by taking a garden hose and running cold water from foot to thigh on each leg, then letting the legs air dry.

WORD TO THE WISE

Fatigue is usually the first sign or symptom that something is wrong in the body. The problem may be a low-grade infection, an inflammation or a reaction to something that shouldn't be in the body, such as chemical food additives. It may be a psychological problem, such as depression over financial problems or an unhappy relationship. Whatever the cause, it is necessary to respond quickly to the fatigue symptom, because if it is allowed to continue, fatigue will lead to exhaustion, inactivity and circulatory inadequacy.

Poor circulation is similar to anemia, which is generally accompanied by weakening of the immune system and vulnerability to disease.

Our first response should be to make sure a balanced food regimen is being used with appropriate food supplements (described in a later chapter).

Our second response should be to take care of the elimination channels by skin brushing; drinking herbal tea such as KB-11 for the kidneys; breathing exercises for the lungs; and colemas to clean out the bowel. Toxins in the bloodstream weaken the heart more than most people realize, and these toxins come from an underactive elimination system. One of the best things we can do for the overburdened heart is to cleanse the bowel with my colema program. A colema is similar to an enema, but much more effective in cleansing the bowel.

When nutrition and tissue cleansing have raised the energy level enough to begin a modest level of exercise—preferably walking—then exercise should be undertaken. Some people start out walking on level ground for a few days. then as they improve, they graduate to a modest grade, perhaps a 3% grade. As they get better at the 3% grade, they graduate again to a steeper slope. I consider this good exercise strategy. When you can handle an exercise easily, increase its difficulty. But talk to your doctor about it first.

Unfortunately, fatigue does not always signal the onset of cardiovascular disease, so it is unwise to settle for a sedentary, underactive lifestyle until fatigue moves in. We should exercise all our lives, at least three or four days a week.

Start early in life to take good care of your body and your body will take good care of you.

CHAPTER 9

STRATEGY FOR BUILDING A HEALTHY HEART

Let's face it—you wouldn't be reading this book if you haven't been living a high-risk lifestyle, as far as your heart is concerned. There must be changes in your life.

Our strategy for building a healthy heart must take into account both what we can do to stop breaking down our heart health and what we can do to help build it up. As a rule, normal heart tissue will repair itself, but it must have a chemically-balanced bloodstream and plenty of blood. We can always tear down our health faster than we can build it up, so the very first step in our strategy must be to change those things in our attitudes, beliefs, jobs, relationships and lifestyles that are breaking down our heart.

The good news about cardiovascular disease and, in particular, atherosclerosis, is that it is not only preventable but reversible. In 1988, Dr. Dean Ornish, assistant clinical professor of medicine at the School of Medicine, University of California at San Francisco, reported the results of a lifestyle change program in which participants used a diet limited to 10% fat, stress management training, moderate exercise and were asked to stop smoking. No cholesterol-lowering drugs were allowed. Not only did the people in the program have a lower blood cholesterol afterward, but they had a measurable reversal of atherosclerosis.

There are risk factors we control in heart disease, and others that we can do nothing about. You can't change risk factors such as age, heredity, previous history of heart disease or being a male. The risk factors you can control are high blood cholesterol, lack of exercise, stress, smoking, high blood pressure and diabetes. The last two factors, high blood pressure and diabetes, require your doctor's participation, but they can be controlled, too.

You need to ask yourself, "What's best for me?" Then make a decision to take the best care possible of your heart, circulatory system and all the rest. Make a mental change first, then the physical changes will follow.

The famous Louis Pasteur once told an audience of doctors to never see a sick patient without asking themselves, "How could I have prevented this from happening?" I have always believed that if doctors did more educating they would do less medicating. Heart disease is a lifestyle disease more than anything else, where prevention is the most effective cure. In the long run, I believe the side effects from drugs do more harm than their primary beneficial effect justifies, so I don't advise using drugs except in emergencies. My approach to building a healthy heart is based upon cooperating with nature and nature's laws.

LET'S REVIEW RISK FACTORS

Many research studies show that cardiovascular disease risk is higher with increasing age, higher in men than women, and higher among the lower-income families than in middle-income or upper-income families. People in the lower-income brackets tend to have diets higher in calories, fats (especially saturated fats), cholesterol and refined carbohydrates (white sugar, white flour, white rice, etc.), and this appears to be where the higher risk is coming from.

I feel the higher risk factor for increasing age is linked with decreasing exercise and dietary imbalance. So, if you are one of those moving into the 50s, 60s and 70s, consider improving your exercise and food habits. Lack of variety in foods is especially evident among the elderly. This must be changed.

FOODS TO AVOID FOR YOUR HEART'S SAKE

It isn't always what we eat that counts, but what we don't eat. There are certain foods that people concerned with preventing or reversing heart disease shouldn't eat, and other foods we shouldn't eat because they lower the rate of function of body systems that support heart health. White flour products don't increase cholesterol or fat levels, but they can slow the bowel and increase toxin level in the blood and lymph. Other foods to avoid are:

Red meat (reduce to once
  a week or less)
Hydrogenated fats
Animal fats
Chocolate
White flour products
Salt
Candy

Shrimp
Milk products
Macadamia nuts
Coconut oil
Ice cream
White sugar products
All fried foods
Rich desserts

Women have less cardiovascular disease than men because the female hormones protect them until menopause. Then they begin catching up with men, especially if lifelong habits such as a high-fat diet loaded with refined carbohydrates is paired with low-exercise motivation. If you are in a rut, get out of it. A rut is a grave with the ends kicked out of it.

FAMILY HISTORY

There is one more set of risk factors we need to look at—family history of heart disease, high blood pressure, diabetes or gout. These are all strong indications of potential heart disease, and I want to discuss them briefly with you.

DIABETES

Diabetes is a blood sugar disorder often related to insulin deficiency because of underactive islands of Langerhans in the pancreas. These tiny endocrine glands imbedded in the pancreas, through their influence on sugar use and storage in the body, apparently influence fat metabolism in the body. The overall effect is to stimulate fat deposits on blood vessel walls. A special diet may bring this under control, or insulin may be needed together with diet.

GOUT

Gout is a type of arthritis involving imbalanced uric acid metabolism in the body. It is favored by excess uric acid in the blood and deposits of uric acid salts in the joints of the hands and feet, and studies show that a significant percentage of those with gout also have cardiovascular disease. Gout, too, responds to diet.

HIGH BLOOD PRESSURE

Of course, hypertension, which is high blood pressure, has been linked with cardiovascular disease for some time. In the past, it has been called hardening of the arteries. I have observed high blood pressure lowered by a combination of dietary measures, stress reduction and tissue cleansing.

The most important reason I have for bringing this up is to point out that the cardiovascular system is dependent for its health and well-being upon every other system in the body—the blood circulation, the lymph, respiration, endocrine glands, digestion, elimination—the whole person. Malfunction in **any** system touches every other system. Gout in the big toe affects the heart, insulin lack from the pancreas affects the heart, damage to the chest brain center in the medulla affects the heart, lack of oxygen affects the heart. Are you getting the idea?

THIS IS IMPORTANT!

You take care of your heart best when you take care of the other 99% of the body surrounding the heart, without neglecting the heart's needs. This is called a wholistic approach to health care.

Every person is born with a constitution made up of mixed inherent weaknesses and strengths, and this mixture differs in each individual. This means that the same diet will not have quite the same effect on any two individuals. A drug that cures one person may kill another. We are all different. Those with a greater number of inherent weaknesses must take better care of themselves to be able to enjoy the same level of health and well-being as those who have fewer inherent weaknesses.

Although we can't control factors like a family history of heart disease (and related diseases), age, sex and affluence, the way we control lifestyle factors, we can **make this information work for us by making a decision to do the best we can with the constitution we have inherited.**

LET'S STOP BREAKING DOWN

What are the risk factors for cardiovascular disease that we can and should control? Let's list them.

Obesity. The solution to obesity is to cut out fatty foods and excess eating, while starting and maintaining a regular exercise program. Get advice from a good nutrition-minded doctor.

Cholesterol. Usually high blood cholesterol comes under control with a low-fat, balanced diet. It is important to realize that lowering our fat intake by 3% causes a 10% lowering of blood cholesterol. (When we cook fatty foods in which cholesterol is initially balanced by lecithin in the raw, uncooked state at heat over 212 degrees F., we destroy the lecithin leaving only the cholesterol. If the cholesterol had been balanced by lecithin, it would not be deposited on arterial walls.)

Hypertension. We may have to cut out coffee (and other caffeine drinks), table salt and take care of our stress problems to reduce high blood pressure.

Diabetes. Proper diet and following your doctor's directions concerning insulin will bring improvement.

Smoking. Find a stop smoking program that fits your needs and take it. Otherwise, just quite cold turkey.

Drinking Alcohol. Cut it out or cut down to two drinks (or two beers or two glasses of wine) daily. If you are an alcohol abuser, talk to your doctor about getting help.

Stress. Working and playing too hard may take their toll on the heart. Work, but don't overwork. Play at what helps you relax. Are you in the right job? Walking, swimming and bicycle riding are great for reducing stress.

Lack of Exercise. Move it or lose it. Walking for one-half an hour to one hour before breakfast is best. You don't have to use the same exercise program that a 20-year-old would use, but you will have to exercise regularly at a level of physical activity that fits your age, ability and diet. It is best to discuss these things with your doctor to make sure you aren't overdoing or underdoing. The older you are, the more good you will get from a sensible level of exercise.

High Blood Level of Uric Acid. If you follow my food regimen, it will drop.

Oral Contraceptives or Post-Menopausal Glandular System Changes should be discussed with your doctor from the perspective of lowering cardiovascular risk.

Friendships. Cultivate healthy friendships and relationships. Stay away from spiteful people.

FOOD REGIMEN: HALF-BUILDING, HALF-CLEANSING

The primary causes of illness and disease are nutritional imbalances and chemical deficiencies on the one hand, and underactive elimination channels resulting in toxic accumulations in the inherently weak tissues on the other hand. For that reason, my food regimen is designed to supply all of the chemical elements, vitamins, enzymes and other nutrients the body needs, but it also supplies plenty of the fiber needed to quicken bowel transit time and avoid constipation. If the bowel is working well, usually the kidneys, skin, lungs and bronchials are eliminating their proper share of waste. To provide balanced nutrition and to avoid underactive waste disposal, my food regimen is half-building and half-cleansing.

The heart gets its oxygen and nutrients from the blood, and if this blood is tainted with toxins, heart tissues will be damaged. How could the blood become tainted with toxins? Toxins are forced into the blood from an underactive bowel, and "unclean" elimination system. To have clean, nutrient rich blood, the diet must be half-building and half-cleansing.

Similarly, the heart will be damaged if there is inadequate oxygen, potassium, glucose and other essential nutrients in the blood. For this reason, we not only need to make sure our foods contain plenty of what the heart needs, but that our digestion is working well and blood circulation is all it should it.

Remember, oxygen is carried by the iron-rich hemoglobin in the blood. If iron is lacking in the diet or our digestive system is unable to assimilate iron to supply the needs of the blood, the heart is adversely affected.

TOO MUCH IS AS BAD AS TOO LITTLE

Too much fat in the diet, too much cholesterol, too much salt and too much sugar may all contribute to the buildup of fatty plaque in the arteries that we call atherosclerosis. My food regimen is balanced to avoid this.

Just as important as a special heart-related food regimen, my food regimen builds healthy blood, nerves, bones, joints, lymph, glands, tissues and organs. Why is this important? It is important because any underfed tissue or organ in the body will drag on the other organs (including the heart), increasing their susceptibility to malfunction and to disease. My food regimen feeds the whole body.

I want to make clear that I believe in cutting out table salt from the diet, but I believe our bodies need food sodium to nourish the digestive system and joints. If a diet is so low in food sodium that the walls of the stomach and small intestine become deficient in sodium reserves, the process of digestion and assimilation will be so disturbed that the heart will be adversely affected. You can't have a good heart together with bad digestion and assimilation. Our bodies need some basic amount of sodium.

EXERCISE TO KEEP THE
HEART AND LUNGS STRONG

The heart is a muscle and like all muscles, it needs exercise—regular exercise—to keep it strong and regular. But, unlike other muscles, the heart is a specialized nerve and muscle organ which needs special care.

Exercise that works out the lungs and the heart is best. Don't overdo, but don't underdo either. Walk at a good clip for half an hour each day. The best time is before breakfast.

Talk to your doctor about the best kinds of exercise and the best program for you.

I believe walking is best. Swimming comes a close second. I have mentioned some wonderful exercises in my chapter on the subject in this book.

PEACE OF MIND

Maybe this should be first instead of last. My mother used to say, "You can lose all your money and you've lost a lot, but if you lose your peace of mind, you'll lose everything." I could write a whole book on this subject alone, but we'll have to settle for less this time.

It is more important than most of us realize to be in a job that we truly feel suits us, to be married to the right person, to have a healthy attitude toward adversity, to have friends who really love us, to keep our finances in order—to do all those things that contribute to our peace of mind.

When we have peace of mind, we have peace of heart, which is true peace. The best rest you can give your heart is the peace that surpasses all understanding, as the Good Book says.

PUTTING IT ALL TOGETHER

Here are my priorities in developing a strategy for a healthy heart.

1. Don't let noncontrollable heart disease risk factors get you down. If your family has a history of heart disease, you can

become the exception. Make up your mind to build a healthy heart.

2. Controllable risk factors. Minimize your risk of heart disease by cutting out or cutting down what harms your heart. Deal with the hardest problem first, such as smoking.

3. Get on a healthy heart food regimen that is half-building and half-cleansing and stay with it.

    a. Nourish the whole body.

    b. Nourish the heart.

    c. Keep your elimination channels open.

    d. Cut out table salt; eat foods high in sodium instead.

4. Exercise every day.

5. Acquire and keep peace of mind.

6. Remember, good health is not a gift, it is earned: you have to work for it.

7. Let your prayer be your work.

INTERESTING HEART FACTS

Heartbeat patterns differ widely; no two are ever alike. The smaller the animal, the faster the heartbeat and, conversely, the larger the animal, the slower the rate. A mouse's heart beats 1,000 times a minute; an elephant's, 35 to 40 beats a minute; a human infant's twice as fast as an adult's; a one-ton white whale's is 15 beats a minute; the average adult human heart—weighing 1/2 pound—records 70 to 72 beats per minute.

CHAPTER 10

BUILDING A HEALTHY HEART
WITH THE RIGHT FOODS

It is difficult to talk about foods any more because so many fad diets have failed to help those who tried them that there is a growing caution and distrust about any new diet. I believe this is a healthy trend in our society. We **should** distrust diets that don't work. It is well to learn from our mistakes.

My healthy heart food regimen is based on over 60 years of experience with clinical nutrition, much of it in a sanitarium setting.

Many times, Dr. V.G. Rocine and his students (like myself) formulated "heart diets" for people with heart disease and those who had been given up by doctors to die. We witnessed many cases of restored heart health in one to three years.

I actually lived with my patients and carefully observed their progress (or lack of it) on a day-to-day basis and week-to-week basis. When we realize that 4,100 Americans have heart attacks every day, which amounts to 123,410 a month, **a reliable diet for building a healthy heart and preventing cardiovascular disease is a must.** Most Americans are getting 40-45% fat in their daily diets, an almost suicidal diet for the heart. My healthy heart food regimen reduces fats and oils in the diet to 20% or less, increases complex carbohydrates (vegetables, fruits and whole grains) to about 65% of the diet and allows about

15% protein. This is within the nutritional guidelines of the National Academy of Sciences.

In the following chapter, I discuss the basics of how food **should** fit into our lives. I think even our attitude to food needs to be changed. Pay close attention as you read this chapter, since the "lessons" in the first part of the chapter are geared to help you make the most out of the Healthy Heart Food Regimen, the sample 7-day menu, and the recipes that follow.

Although I have seen many of my patients "outgrow" their symptoms by right living and right food habits, even in the early days of my practice, I have continued to improve my nutritional program as I made new discoveries and developed new insights into the way foods fit into the health-building process. I have been able to help many patients with heart ailments.

LESSON ONE—HOW TO EAT

Everyone you and i know is able to put food in his or her mouth, but that doesn't mean they know how to eat. Some people eat so fast you could almost believe they were inhaling their food. Others pick at what is on their plate, eating the meat and potatoes and pushing the vegetables aside. To get the most good from what we eat, we need to reconsider some basic mealtime wisdom and adopt a few guidelines to put that wisdom to work.

Those who bolt down their food will need to learn how to slow down and enjoy their food more. Parents accustomed to disciplining their children at the dinner table or arguing at mealtimes will need to learn that they are seriously impairing their own digestion and assimilation as well as that of their children. Mealtimes must be pleasant to get the most out of our food. People who read or watch TV while they eat are allowing their gland and nervous systems to be sidetracked from the main business at hand—getting the best from their food.

If not entirely comfortable in mind and body, don't eat. It is best to eat when your appetite is keen for simple, plain foods. If this means you have to cut out between meal snacking, then do it. Skip meals if you are emotionally upset, chilled, overheated, in pain, ill or just plain not hungry. Trust your body's food and hunger cues. You don't have to eat every meal.

We find that it is very important to eat slowly, enjoy each mouthful of food and stop when our hunger is satisfied. This may involve leaving some food on your plate, saying no to second helpings and having dessert only once in a while. But if our meals are balanced, we should always eat some of everything on the plate.

Look at your food as you eat it. Notice the smells. Savor the taste. Don't forget to compliment the cook. If you have tended to rush through mealtimes in the past, put down your fork between bites. We need to stir our digestive juices and stimulate our brain and nerves to prepare our digestive system to respond appropriately to what we are eating.

This way of eating not only makes each meal a special, enjoyable occasion, but brings about the most complete digestion possible for each individual.

LESSON TWO—PHILOSOPHY FOR PEACEFUL DIGESTION

It is well known that our emotions and moods create a climate in which digestion responds for the better or for the worse. In my experience, it is possible for a person to adopt a philosophy toward many of life's experiences that increases peace of mind and equilibrium. This is good, very good, for the heart and digestion.

To begin with, we all need to learn to be more thankful about the many good things that come into our lives and to be willing to bless people, especially those who are hard for us to like. Make up your mind that you are going to forgive and forget every wrong done to you and be willing to apologize to those you have wronged. Try to avoid being a critic, judge, advisor or corrector of others and their mistakes. Let them live and learn, like you did, from their own mistakes.

Learn to live in harmony with your fellow man, nature and changing times. All three will be here at least as long as we will.

Accept decisions once they are made and avoid crying over spilled milk. Make the best of circumstances, even if they are not what you would have preferred.

Avoid gossip or any unnecessary uncomplimentary remarks about anyone. Gossip is an insult to the dignity of the human soul.

Spend 10 minutes a day meditating on how to be a better person. The mind initiates and the body follows.

If your conversation with others, in general, tends to be mainly negative, turn it around until it becomes mainly positive. Be patient. It takes time to get out of a negative frame of reference and to become more positive and uplifting. Your heart will love you for it.

Work out your problems in the morning when you are fresh and creative. Don't take them to bed with you. Don't let the sun go down on your anger.

LESSON THREE—KITCHEN PRINCIPLES

Don't fry foods; use heated oils or use concentrated vegetable oils (except for a little in salad dressings). Remember, frying food, whether pan frying or deep fat frying, saturates the food (and its batter coating, if any) with fat. You get enough fats and oils in the lean meat, chicken, fish, vegetables, nuts and seeds you eat to meet your body's needs.

Bake, broil or roast the meat, chicken and fish you eat, as a healthier alternative to frying. The idea is to limit your overall intake of fat calories to less than 20% of your total daily calories. You may want to have two or more fully vegetarian meals per week, especially if you have been a heavy meat eater in the past.

Cook in stainless steel, low heat cooking utensils. Steaming vegetables in a steamer is a reasonable alternative. Avoid cooking at high heat as much as possible, since it causes an undesirable chemical change in food.

Use as few refined foods (white flour, white sugar, white polished rice) as possible. They are nutritionally deficient. Substitute vegetable seasonings from the health food store for salt. Learn to use individual herbs and combinations of herbs for seasoning, rather than salt. Table salt is refined at high heat and has a chemical in it to make it pour easily. If you must use salt, use evaporated sea salt.

LESSON FOUR—FOLLOW A SOUND
FOOD PHILOSOPHY

I use whole foods as much as possible as the heart of my food program. Whole foods contain all the vitamins, minerals, enzymes and nutrients that nature originally put in them. They are in the right balance, in the right ratios to one another for proper use by the body. By whole foods, I mean foods like eggs, raw seeds, potatoes with the skins, whole grains—foods capable of reproducing life. They have the "life factors" in them: enzymes, prostaglandins, combinations of vitamins and minerals that work well together in the body. In contrast to whole foods, refined white flour, white rice, powdered eggs, peeled potatoes and packaged commercial breakfast cereals are all examples of foods that were once whole, but have had a nutritionally significant part of the original food removed. The nutritional value is much less.

Please notice, I am not saying that all foods from which something is removed should be cast aside. We can't eat pineapple skins or cores, but the fruit still is nutritionally valuable. We don't eat carrot tops, nut shells, avocado skins or seeds, chicken bones or fish heads. Only part of these foods is conveniently and practically edible. But, in general, we should use as much of each food we buy and prepare as possible, to get the greatest nutritional value from them.

Closely related to the idea of using whole foods (for their higher nutritional value) is the principle of using pure foods as much as possible. A pure food is a food to which nothing has been added: no preservatives, no artificial flavors, no texture enhancers, no thickeners, no salt, no sugar, no pickling agent and no other substances. Many food additives have been declared carcinogenic and illegal in recent years, which shows a significant level of risk in the original selection process. This is a good reason to avoid them as much as possible.

I believe in using foods that are pure, whole, natural and fresh. Sprayed foods are not pure. Foods containing chemical additives are not pure. Pickled, salted or processed foods are not pure. No food is really pure unless it is grown in soil that is not contaminated by manufactured chemical fertilizer, pesticide sprays or other chemicals. Pure **means** nothing added by man.

As of this writing, red dye No. 5 has been declared illegal for use in lipstick, candy and pill coatings. Red No. 5 has been controversial for many years, as some consumer groups insisted it was carcinogenic and manufacturers using it declared it was not. Finally, the Federal government has declared that it is carcinogenic, based on a laboratory test in which a certain percentage of rats that ingested the dye developed thyroid cancer.

Manufacturers select chemical additives which will save them money (by prolonging the shelf life of the product) or increase their profits (by making the product more attractive). This means that the food industry tests additives for such qualities as effectiveness in preserving a food from bacterial decomposition or spoilage, flavor or flavor enhancement, color or color enhancement, thickening, improvement of texture, bleaching and other purposes. The health and safety of the consumer is primarily reduced only to a defensive consideration in the profit picture. Obviously, if some additive in a food product makes a lot of people sick, no one will buy it. But, if the additive takes 20 years to cause health problems, who will ever find out?

I have had many patients at my Ranch who were allergic to various chemical sprays or food additives. It is possible that one day we will discover that chemical food additives have contributed far more to major health problems than we now know. Many products are loaded with salt, which always increases the cardiovascular risk to the consumer. Why take a chance? Stick to pure foods as much as possible.

Lastly, my food philosophy is to use only natural foods as much as possible. "Natural" means as found in nature. A cucumber is natural; a pickled cucumber is not. A whole grain of wheat is natural; a milled grain of wheat is not. We could debate the fine points, but I would consider whole wheat flour natural from a practical standpoint, even though man has changed its form. I do not consider flour made from milled wheat as natural because it is missing the bran, the germ and the natural oils, vitamins and minerals in the germ layer. Saccharine is an unnatural, artificially manufactured "food." An organically-grown, tree-ripened apricot is natural.

This is the basis of my approach to nutrition: Food must be whole, pure, fresh and natural. This is my basic food philosophy.

INTRODUCING
MY HEALTHY HEART FOOD REGIMEN

Now we are ready to get into my Healthy Heart Food Regimen. To start with, we should have 6 vegetables, 2 fruits, 1 good starch and 1 good protein, at least 5 out of the 7 days of the week. As I have suggested before, it is all right to have two completely vegetarian days each week. (These can be either strict vegetarian or you may include eggs and milk products for the protein.)

Why should we have this particular proportion of foods? There are several reasons.

First of all, most people get too few vegetables and fruits in their diet. The vegetables and fruits provide most of the vitamins, minerals, enzymes, fiber and some of the carbohydrates needed in our bodies. Also 6 vegetables and 2 fruits in the proper amounts will make up 80% of our daily diet. (The USDA recommends only two servings of fruit and three of vegetables.) This amount of fruits and vegetables is a deliberate decision on my part, because our bodies need 80% alkaline-forming foods and 20% acid-forming foods. We need the alkaline salts to neutralize the acidic wastes in the body. The alkaline salts of calcium, potassium and sodium do most of the acid neutralizing, but salts of magnesium, manganese and others also help. Proteins, starches and sugars are nearly all acid-forming foods. Our single starch and single protein, again in the right proportion by weight, makes up 20% of the daily diet.

Why do I recommend the 80%-to-20% alkaline/acid ratio? The normal pH of the blood is 7.35 to 7.45 on a scale of 0 (completely acid) to 14 (completely alkaline), which means that our blood is slightly alkaline (7 is in the middle). A pH of 7.35 to 7.45 is necessary for many of the chemical reactions which take place at the level of tissue and cell metabolism. To stabilize this alkaline/acid level in the body requires 80% alkaline foods in the diet to neutralize the predominantly acid metabolic wastes and keep the blood slightly alkaline.

We need the protein for tissue repair and maintenance and the starch for energy. Enough fats and oils are found in the protein, vegetables and whole grains (starches) to meet the lipid needs of the body metabolism.

The U.S. government says the average American diet is only 20% fruit and vegetables and nearly 45% fat. I estimate the average diet in this country is at least 50%-to-60% acid-forming foods.

WHAT DOES THIS MEAN FOR THE HEART?

It means that large amounts of alkaline salts will be used up in neutralizing acid wastes. This can deplete the heart of its potassium needed to neutralize the metabolic wastes produced in the heart muscle. This weakens the heart muscle and may increase its vulnerability to heart attack and other problems.

I have always believed in the need for a variety of fruits and vegetables in the diet. My aunt has plenty of vegetables with her meals, but she always has only peas and carrots. That's not variety. The purpose of variety is to make sure we are getting a sufficient array of vitamins, minerals and other nutrients to meet **all** the special nutrient needs of the different organs, glands and tissues in the body, *leaving none deficient in any chemical element*. This is best accomplished by including as large a variety of foods as possible in our food regimen.

The average American diet is 63% wheat, milk and sugar: 29% wheat products, 25% milk products and 9% sugar products. This is a very unhealthy situation. Wheat and milk should make up no more than 6% of our total daily diet, but if you have been a heavy wheat or milk user, you may want to cut them out of your food regimen altogether.

In short, the average American diet is dangerous to the heart, while my Healthy Heart Food Regimen is a reasonable step toward halting the progress of cardiovascular disease and possibly beginning to reverse the abnormal deposits and tissue abnormalities.

DR. JENSEN'S HEALTHY HEART
FOOD REGIMEN

I will present the basic food regimen first, then fill it in with specific food and menu recommendations.

Before Breakfast. Upon arising and half hour before breakfast, have a glass of unsweetened natural fruit juice or a teaspoon of liquid chlorophyll in a glass of warm water or a broth and lecithin drink made of one teaspoon vegetable broth powder and one tablespoon of lecithin granules dissolved in a glass of warm water.

Brush your skin for 5 minutes with a natural bristle, long-handled brush (available at many health food stores).

Take half an hour brisk walk or do other exercises, as approved by your doctor. You may do sniff-breathing exercises as you walk by inhaling a breath in four short vigorous sniffs, exhale in one long breath and repeat this for five minutes. (For best results, use sniff-breathing exercises before lunch and before dinner.)

Lastly, take your shower or bath. If you shower, start with warm water and gradually turn to cooler water until your breath quickens. Do not shower immediately upon getting out of bed.

Our mealtime philosophy is, "Eat like a prince or princess at breakfast, a king or queen at lunch and a pauper at dinner." If you have difficulty sleeping at night, try having your protein at another meal and have a starch and vegetable only. Heart experts now say it is best not to have wine (or other alcoholic beverage) with meals. If you are taking a B-Complex vitamin supplement, take it at breakfast or lunch, since B-Complex can interfere with sleep.

Foods are made of the chemical elements, and the heart especially needs potassium, silicon, iron, calcium, magnesium and zinc in the foods we eat. If we are dealing with cardiovascular disease, it may be well to go on a short cleansing fast or diet before trying to feed the heart with the foods it truly needs. Even the heart may have toxins imbedded in its muscle tissue or attached fatty tissue, and it is best to get rid of as much of this as we can.

Those with heart troubles should also use the sodium foods to neutralize metabolic acids in the lymph and bloodstream, to keep them from irritating the heart as they pass through in the blood. The dried goat whey product called Capri Mineral Whey is high in food sodium and is an easy supplement to take. Capri Mineral Whey may be obtained from Mt. Capra Cheese, 279 SW 9th Street, Chehalis, WA 98532.

CHEMICAL ELEMENTS IN DRIED GOAT WHEY
(Micrograms per gram)

Boron	5.20	Sodium	4200.00
Barium	3.10	Phosphorus	6100.00
Calcium	2900.00	Sulfur	850.00
Chromium	0.52	Selenium	1.40
Copper	0.99	Tin	3.80
Iron	6.60	Thallium	2.20
Potassium	2500.00	Vanadium	0.14
Magnesium	1200.00	Zinc	2.70

Experiments have shown that increasing the potassium chloride availability (just a little) slowed the heart's rate and force, while increasing the calcium chloride tended to increase the same things. Other heart salts, taken from foods, must be present for the normal working of the heart. The heart can't get by on simply any chemical elements.

When the iron in the blood is low, the pulse may become soft—almost imperceptible. The reason is that when iron is low, oxygen is also low. Since the heart needs a great deal of oxygen, lack of this important element seriously handicaps the heart. It slows down. When the blood iron is normal and calcium is abundant in the blood, the pulse is large, full, long and slow. Calcium gives expansive power to the heart. Calcium deficiency is indicated by a "nervous pulse." Potassium deficiency produces spasmodic contractions of the heart.

As long as we supply the chemical elements needed by the heart and its activities, we have nothing to fear. A heart "that never stops" as long as we live must be supplied with the right food chemicals. But, the principle life impulse is in the medulla.

The heartbeat is influenced by many agents—worry, fear, joy, gloom, drugs, diets, drinks, heavy metals, acids in the body, gases in the blood, stomach gas presses on the heart, breathing, work rate, staying up late, loss of sleep, heat, cold, athletics, age, body position, oxygen in the air, altitude, blood pressure, air pressure and others. Nicotine decreases the heart rate. Caffeine increases it. Nothing benefits the heart as much as the proper foods.

Breakfast. Have fruit in season. Dried fruit, reconstituted by soaking in boiling water, may be substituted. Health drink, such as herbal tea or a non-citrus fruit juice or vegetable broth drink. Whole grain cereal or muesli. Choose from yellow cornmeal, brown rice, millet, rye or oats (rolled oats or steel-cut oats). Cook whole grain cereal over very low heat, tightly covered. The best way is to soak it overnight in boiling water in a wide-mouth thermos. You may substitute one or two eggs, boiled or poached only, up to three times per week. Cut down protein at lunch or dinner accordingly. You may use a coffee substitute.

10 A.M. It is best to avoid mid-morning snacks and take a relaxation break instead. If you desire, however, you may have a vegetable juice drink or broth drink.

Lunch. Emphasis at lunch should be on a big salad, with mixed greens. Be creative and use as many leafy greens and vegetable ingredients as you can. Do yourself a favor and get a copy of my book, *Dr. Jensen's Real Soup and Salad Book*, and you'll look forward to lunches as never before. Avoid filling up on protein first. *Always start with the salad or other vegetables.* Remember to dilute salad dressings and use them sparingly, since they can be an inconspicuous but high source of calories. If you buy salad dressings, *read the labels to see if salt and other chemical additives are used.* It is better to make your own dressings. If sugar is called for, use honey or a fruit concentrate syrup instead. If salt is called for, use a vegetable or herbal seasoning instead. You may wish to have a cup of soup with your lunch, and your protein can be part of your salad—such as cold chicken or turkey cut into bite-sized pieces, cold precooked tuna or salmon, sliced hard-boiled eggs and so forth, or you can have your protein separate from the salad. You may wish to have a hot cooked vegetable or two with your salad and protein.

3 P.M. Snack time. Health drink. Fruit such as small apple, pear or banana. Or have two Ry-Krisp crackers with sesame butter. Keep it low-cal, saltless and sugarless.

Dinner. Here's where we must be careful, because going to bed soon after an evening meal encourages weight gain and higher blood cholesterol, two no-no's for heart health. Why?

Because when you sleep, your metabolism slows down, less energy is burned, and your brain tells your digestion and body systems to convert everything that can't be kept in the blood to glycogen or fat and store it. That's why I say, "Eat like a pauper at dinner." The best thing you can do for yourself is to make a decision *to eat lightly at every dinner and love it!*

Soup and salad dinners with a baked potato or a nice hunk of baked squash can be very satisfying. Cooked greens like spinach, chard or mustard greens are good with an evening meal. Steamed brown rice or wild rice (or a mix of the two) with herbal seasonings is delicious. **Note:** Watch the amount of butter or margarine used on a baked potato, yam, sweet potato, rice, vegetables, etc. Try using a little low-fat yogurt on vegetables after sprinkling with vegetable broth powder, instead of using butter or margarine. Use as little concentrated oils, butter and margarine as possible in your food regimen.

Before Bedtime. Skin brush with a natural bristle brush for five minutes.

SUMMARY OF
HEALTHY HEART REGIMEN STRATEGY

1. Before breakfast have a health drink, skin brush, exercise 1/2 hour, sniff breathing, shower.
2. Breakfast. Emphasis on juice, fruit and cooked whole grain cereal or muesli.
3. 10 a.m. Rest or have juice or broth.
4. Lunch. Emphasis on salad and protein.
5. 3 p.m. Snack or health drink.
6. Dinner. Emphasis on salad, cooked vegetables, starch.
7. Before bed. Skin brush.

RECOMMENDED SUPPLEMENTS
FOR A HEALTHY HEART

Liquid chlorophyll
Wheat germ
Vitamin E
Brown rice
Cereals
Vitamins B, B-12, iron
Selenium
Tsp honey in glass of water
Apple cider vinegar in dressings
Hawthorne berry tea

SAMPLE MENUS AND RECIPES

My Healthy Heart Food Regimen is deliberately low in concentrated fats and oils (both saturated and unsaturated, animal and vegetable); cholesterol; dairy products; refined carbohydrates; salt; red meat; and all foods and condiments associated with cardiovascular disease. My Healthy Heart Regimen is deliberately high in vegetables and fruits that offer biochemical mineral and vitamin groups associated with cardiovascular health and well-being, such as potassium, calcium, magnesium, iodine, iron, vitamins A, B-Complex, C,

D, E, niacin (B-3) and rutin. Natural fiber found in all fruits, vegetables, whole grains, raw nuts and seeds, speeds up bowel activity which eliminates more cholesterol and triglycerides rather than giving them increased time to be absorbed through the bowel wall. We need 30 grams of fiber daily.

Fiber Content of Some Common Foods

Food	Grams of Fiber
Apple, 1 small	1.0
Asparagus, 1/2 cup	2.8
Banana, 1 medium	0.5
Beans, lima, 1/4 cup	1.8
Beans, string, 3/4 cup	1.0
Beets, diced, 1/2 cup	0.8
Beet greens, cooked, 1/2 cup	1.3
Bread, whole wheat, 1 slice	2.1
Bread, white, 1 slice	0.2
Broccoli, cooked, 1/2 cup	1.7
Brussels sprouts, 1/2 cup	2.7
Carrots, cooked, 3/4 cup	1.0
Cereals:	
All Bran, 1/2 cup	24.9
Cream of Wheat, cooked, 1/2 cup	trace
Oatmeal, cooked, 3/4 cup	0.2
Oat bran, 1/2 cup dry	7.2
Rolled oats, cooked, 1/2 cup	0.8
Shredded wheat biscuit, 1/2 cup	10.2
Eggplant, 1/2 cup diced, cooked	2.5
Honeydew melon, 1 med. wedge	1.3
Lettuce, 1/6 head	1.4
Orange, 1 med.	3.0
Pear, 1 med.	3.0
Peas, fresh green, 3/4 cup	2.0
Prunes, 6 med., 2 tbsp juice	0.8
Raspberries, red, 3/4 cup	3.0
Spinach, 1/2 cup boiled	5.7
Strawberries, fresh, 2/3 cup	1.4
Tomato, 1 med. raw	2.0

NOTE: These figures are based on several sources, each with a potentially wide variation in the actual fiber content of the different foods. This chart is merely to acquaint the reader with the approximate fiber content of some foods.

SOUPS AND BROTHS FOR
HEART-BUILDING IN LEAN PEOPLE

Chicken bone broth	Lobster broth
Crab broth	Oyster broth
Clam broth	Broth from greens
Sea crab broth	Fruit soup
King crab broth	Milk soup

Broth from cooked fresh bones (no fat) with greens added.

The heart broths are for those who don't have the proper blood salts. These broths are not meant for persons who are in relatively good health. They are intended to save a lean person's life when heart trouble is present. This is bringing him back to the place where he can build up his body as quickly as possible.

A broth is not a soup. A broth should be a strong decoction, cooked long and slowly, so the vitamins and minerals are not altered or reduced. A broth should simmer slowly. Greens may be added to the broth. Greens are high in potassium, the main chemical element.

There are times when a concentrated source of iron is needed, and it can be obtained from meat, poultry and fish. When iron is sufficient, we don't have to look to the meat sources but we can look to other foods for an abundance of vitamins, minerals and enzymes.

Vital food juices such as carrot juice mixed with raw goat milk make a wonderful broth or liquid drink. This will bring you many of the food properties you need.

If you are going to use any of the meats, they should be cooked rare and never burned. Never eat any healthy meals.

Heavy meals put a burden on the heart. We must eat small meals and eat often. We find that fish contains oils that reduce the risk of heart attack. Fish have properties unknown to the vegetable kingdom. These are times when we need to go to the meat, chicken and fish for concentrated food values. The vegetarian can get some of these values from supplements such as chlorella, tofu (a soy protein), sea algae and other specialty foods and supplements.

GREENS FOR HEART BUILDING IN THE LEAN MAN

Celery heart	Clover buds (salads)
Alfalfa buds (salads)	Fruit blossoms (salads)
Dill	Young lettuce
Crisp lettuce	Young winter lettuce
Celery cabbage	Corn parsley
Chive	Common parsley
Mint	Young romaine
Cabbage sprouts	Tender Swiss chard
Peppermint	Tender spinach, steamed

One salad eaten each day, made of many salad ingredients, with egg-yolk dressing or egg-whit dressing, cream or coconut cream dressing, to supply food material for the internal glands, also to supply building material to the heart is a good habit for the health of the heart.

VEGETABLES FOR HEART BUILDING
IN THE LEAN MAN

Artichokes	Asparagus tops
Corn on cob	Kohlrabi
Muskmelon	Okra and tomatoes

Sweet green peas
Hearts of gold melon
Cooked beets
Head lettuce
Steamed onions
Watermelon
Winter melon
Georgia rattlesnake melon

Cantaloupe
Casaba
Eggplant
Okra
Squash
Globe artichokes
Pumpkin

FRUITS TO SELECT FROM

Avocado
Blueberry juice
Blackcap juice
Dewberry sauce
Fresh figs
Green figs
Mangoes
Ripe olives
Papaya sauce
Yellow plums
Persimmons
Stewed pears
Prune sauce

Blackberry juice
Black cherries
Black currant sauce
Dewberry juice
Black sun-dried figs
Grape sauce (no sugar)
Mulberries
Papaya
Satsuma plums
Fig sauce
Huckleberries and sauce
Elderberry juice

CEREALS

Whole rice meal muffins
Rye meal bread
Whole rye meal
Coconut, rice meal muffins
other spices
Raisins/dry zante currants
in breads, muffins

Whole rice meal bread
Steel-cut oatmeal
Barley meal loaf
Hot tomatoes on hot Caraway,
bread

DAIRY PRODUCTS

Goat buttermilk

Beaten egg white in milk

Goat cream

Coconut cream

Beaten egg white w/angelfood cake made w/whole wheat flour

Poached eggs

Milk toast

Goat milk whey

Goat cottage cheese

Roquefort cheese

Goat butter

Baked custard

Egg yolk shakes

Fresh goat milk

Eggs scrambled lightly in milk

Milk soup

PUDDINGS

Whole rice fruit

Custard

Bread

Milk

Banana

Sago (rarely)

SWEETS

We should be careful to avoid most sweets, especially white sugar and candies or syrups made from it.

> It is wise for a lean man with heart trouble to eat sparingly of butter, coconut, puddings, milk, also of cereals, because such foods are acid-forming, and may make the heart tissues and the stomach more acid, if over indulged. Cut out citrus fruits. We should drink between meals, never at meals, though hot broths are favorable at meals.

Most of us should try to grow as much of our own foods as we can. Vegetable gardens can be easily planted and maintained to our great advantage. We should try to get eggs from healthy, free-roaming hens. We should have a couple of milk goats. If we are going to build a new heart, we have to stay away from foods that are not going to repair, rebuild and take care of us. The packaged, processed foods are the ones that can make us sick. Be very careful in your food purchases. Health does not care for itself. We find that the wrong diet undermines the heart. The correct diet rebuilds the heart.

HEART-BUILDING FOODS
FOR OVERWEIGHT PEOPLE

Fresh crabs
Crab broth
Steamed heart
Calf liver
Rice bran raisin muffins
Wild cherry juice
Sun-dried olives
Baked fish roe
Cottage cheese w/pineapple
German sauerkraut muffins
Veal joint jelly
Salad w/egg white, lemon
 dressing
Shredded wheat biscuit w/
 dried Zante currants

Fresh lettuce
Romaine
Steamed kidney
Lobster broth
Crab meat
Steamed spinach
Celery broth
Roquefort cheese
Steamed onions
Steamed smelt
Whole rice meal, steel-
 cut muffins w/Zante
 currants
Dwarf nettle salad

You may want to discuss the use of these foods with a nutrition-minded doctor. Otherwise, use them as an adjunct to my regular heart diet for a month.

HEART TONIC

A wonderful heart tonic may be made of raw meat juice and milk made alkaline with egg white, water and juice from celery heart, (or mixed with juice pressed out of romaine, celery, dandelion, dill, parsley or dwarf nettles.

The heart muscle is always acid in overweight people with heart trouble, but often also in lean people with the same problem.

THE SECOND HEART-BUILDING DIET PERIOD FOR OVERWEIGHT PEOPLE

Those on this diet will have to have the gas driver supplements and alkalinizers. We find that we have to use such drinks, teas, tonics and foods that help to overcome acidity and gas that may disturb the health, vigor and freedom of the heart. In the blood and tissues, we can find dissolved gases. We don't want any gases that interfere with the health of the heart.

SOUPS AND BROTHS FOR OVERWEIGHT PEOPLE

Bone joint broth, fat removed Lobster broth
Chicken bone broth   Crab broth
Clam broth   Eggshell broth (2 doz
Vegetable broth (6-12   shells cooked for 2 hr)
 different greens)

These broths feed the heart nerves, the heart brain and steady the heartbeat, if continued for some time. All broths are prepared by simmering. All these broths are important, though some contain heart and nerve food in greater abundance. For overweight people, the broth should be concentrated or simmered down to a cup, 3/4ths full.

MEAT AND FISH FOR OVERWEIGHT PEOPLE

Green turtle
Broiled chicken
Tender broiled ham
Crab meat
Smoked haddock
Veal joint jelly
Broiled wild game
Kidney
Black bass

Smoked salmon
Smoked herring
Shrimp
Smoked halibut
Young liver
Boiled perch
Heart
Frog legs
Shad

GREENS AND VEGETABLES
FOR OVERWEIGHT PEOPLE

Chives
Chicory
Dandelion broth
Celery broth
Dwarf nettles
Sage
Beet tops
Collards
Thyme
Spearmint
Radish leaves
Lamb's lettuce

Chard
Chervil
German sauerkraut
Leek greens
Parsley
Shallot
Sugar beet leaves
White carrots
Cress
Peppermint
Kale broth
Early curled lettuce

Big Boston lettuce	May king lettuce
White lettuce	Yellow beets, sparingly
Broccoli	Red grated carrots
Steamed savoy cabbage	Panama rhubarb
Leeks	White young radishes
lack young radishes	Red young radishes
White steamed onions	Swiss chard
Yellow tomatoes	Burbank tomatoes
Fresh lima beans w/lemon juice, egg white dressing	String beans w/lemon juice, egg white dressing

> The greens and vegetables here that are high in potassium, iron, sodium, sulphur, calcium, and those that are bitter in nature, build better blood. They tone the feeble heart and promote elimination regardless of their moisture, fat and carbohydrate content. The contents of fats, sugar, starch, protein and moisture are often low in most greens and in a great many vegetables. We find that the greens taken with dried goat whey always reduce the weight of the body. A high-chlorine diet dehydrates the body or attracts water from the body.

THE HIGHEST CHLORINE FOODS

Seafoods are the richest source of chlorine, followed by raw goat milk. Chlorine-containing foods are listed below. (* denotes highest foods in chlorine.)

Asparagus	Horseradish, raw
Avocados	Jerusalem artichoke
Bananas	Kale
Beans	Kelp
Beechnuts	Kohlrabi

Beets	Lean meats
Blackberries	Leeks
Brazil nuts	Lentils
Breadfruit	Lettuce, leaf, sea
Brussels sprouts	Mangoes
Cabbage	Oats
Carrots	Onions, dry
Cauliflower	Parsnips
Celery	Peaches
Cheeses	Peas
Chicory	Pineapple
Chickpeas, dried	Potatoes w/skins
Chives	Radishes
Coconut	Raisins
Corn	Red raspberries
Cowpeas, dried	Rutabaga
Cucumbers	Seafoods
Dandelion greens	Sauerkraut
Dates	Spinach
Dock (sorrel)	Strawberries
Eggplant	Sunflower seeds
Endive	Sweet potatoes
Figs	Tomatoes
Filberts	Turnips
*Fish	Veal joint broth
Fowl	Watercress
*Goat milk, raw	Watermelon
Guava	White beans, dried

We find that taking the foods listed will help protect the heart, as well as cleansing the body at the tissue level.

On a diet of foods containing sufficient sodium, potassium, chlorine and iron, carbohydrates are better utilized and excess moisture is kept from the heart tissue, resulting in real tissue building, not water logging or fatty buildup. Overweight men and women should not have heavy meals, and not much food at each meal. Overweight people are the ones that have the highest risk of heart disease. They should eat small meals.

Divide meals up into five small meals daily. Breakfast should include a whole grain cereal and fruit. The mid-morning meal might be a slice of goat cheese with Ry-Krisp, and a glass of carrot juice. Lunch might consist of a large, raw garden salad with plenty of leafy, green vegetables, a bowl of barley-kale soup and a rice cracker spread with raw sesame seed butter. The mid-afternoon meal could be a baked potato, celery sticks and lemon grass tea. Dinner should be something like a small piece of fish and a rainbow salad (green, leafy vegetables, cutup scallions, parsley, tomatoes, grated carrots, grated turnip, grated beets, sprinkled with finely-ground almonds and a tablespoon of dried goat whey, a dried goat whey food supplement high in food sodium, potassium, chlorine, magnesium and many trace elements); a cooked vegetable like green beans or corn may be added, and a health drink, like goat milk or oat straw tea. (A tablespoon of dried goat whey should also be taken at the breakfast meal, in a cup of hot water.) No foods should be taken two hours before bedtime.

FRUIT FOR OVERWEIGHT PEOPLE

Stewed sun-dried apples	Dried Zante currants
Grapefruit	Limes
Dried olives (have daily)	Revived dried peaches
Strawberry sauce	Wild strawberries
Pineapple sauce	Sun-dried prunes
Tangerines	Black currants
Nectarines	Florida oranges
White currant sauces	Mandarins
Pineapple	Pomegranates
Quince	White raspberries
Black raspberries	Home-cooked fruit
Any sun-dried, subacid fruit (no sugar)	Twice cooked sun-dried pears

When I say "cooked," "fresh," "subacid," "no sugar," "dried olives," "sun dried," I mean exactly that. Sun-dried olives are the highest food in potassium. You can dry them yourself or you can get them from an Italian or Greek store. They are called "sun-dried olives." You can revive them by soaking them in warm water overnight. Add a touch of olive oil, if you wish, to give them an oily taste. I never recommend factory-dried, sulfured fruit. Such fruit could ruin the heart. That is why I say "sun dried" or "home-dried fruit." A sick heart cannot tolerate chemicalized foods.

CEREALS FOR OVERWEIGHT PEOPLE

Steel-cut oatmeal, well cooked. Bran muffins made with dried Zante currants. Whole rice meal muffins with dried Zante currants, and well spiced. Muffins made of Kellogg's starchless bran are excellent. Imported Ry-Krisp (used sparingly). Have no wheat.

I find that most cereals are not favorable for an overweight person. We should have less of the bread, especially. Substitute rice cakes or rye crackers which come from Sweden and Norway.

DRINKS FOR OVERWEIGHT PEOPLE

Blackberry juice
Black currant juice
Greens
Broths, as recommended
Peppermint tea
Saffron tea
Sage tea/clam broth, mixed
Grapefruit
Lemonade (hot, no sugar)
Celery juice
Wild cherry juice
Egg shell broth
Parsley tea
Raw goat buttermilk
Skim milk
Grapefruit/ginger ale
Limeade (hot, no sugar)
Bone broth

When the overweight person gets thirsty, no drink more favorable than hot limeade or hot, sour lemonade can be found. He may not like such a drink, but it favors his heart and health. The overweight man should not drink too much liquid or it will be hard on his heart.

DAIRY PRODUCTS FOR OVERWEIGHT PEOPLE

Beaten egg white on salads   Goat buttermilk
Goat milk cottage cheese   Egg white shake in skim
Imported Swiss cheese (little)   milk, well beaten
Skim milk

If we are going through a heart-building program, we should leave out delicacies, pies, sweets, cakes and so forth. We cannot build a good heart on puddings and so forth. We must have foods that are going to rebuild the cell structure. Drinks and foods highly important in the foregoing heart diet are those containing sodium chloride, potassium and calcium. They are preferable and should be eaten often. We have gotten to the place where it is fashionable even for men to cook. We consider the wise cook to be a kitchen doctor. The health of his or her family is in the cook's hands. A wise cook can add many years of quality life to a person, while an ignorant or uncaring cook may lead people to an early grave. I must tell you, I am opposed to the use of concentrated fats and oils (except in a little salad dressing) outside of the food. We should have only the fats that come with the food. Our bodies can take the fats in cream, in avocados, in coconuts, in sesame seeds and in Missouri black walnuts because it is accompanied by nutrients that help our bodies utilize the fats properly. We all need a little of the fats in our diet, but it should come from the foods.

119

A WEEK OF HEART-FRIENDLY MENUS

Day 1, Breakfast

Apple juice, 8 oz; oatmeal, 1 cup cooked and topped with honey or fruit concentrate, 1 tbsp; half cantaloupe, slice of cornbread; herbal tea or coffee substitute.

10 am Snack

Carrot juice, 8 oz.

Lunch

Lemon grass herbal tea, 8 oz; large garden salad topped with grated turnip, grated beet and finely-ground almonds; broiled halibut steak or fillet, 8 oz; steamed zucchini and pearl onions; strawberries and low-fat natural yogurt, if desired.

3 pm Snack

V-8 juice, 8 oz, and a slice of rye bread with sesame butter.

Dinner

Large yam baked (in foil), small garden salad topped with grated carrots; cooked peas and carrots; steamed millet, Chico-San rice crackers, peppermint tea.

No Before-Bed Snacks.

Day 2, Breakfast

Prune juice, 4 oz; cracked rye cereal, 1 cup cooked and topped with honey or maple syrup; poached egg; 2 Ry-Krisp crackers; comfrey-fenugreek tea.

10 am Snack

Red delicious apple, small.

Lunch

Peppermint tea, 8 oz; large garden salad topped with grated parsnips, grated carrot and finely-ground sesame seed (hulled); London broil, 8 oz; steamed grated beets topped with low-fat yogurt or 2 tbsp sour cream.

3 pm Snack

Raw celery and carrot sticks, 6 each.

Dinner

Baked potato topped with vegetable broth powder, low-fat yogurt and chives; a small garden salad; cooked green beans; steamed millet.

Day 3, Breakfast

Grape juice, 8 oz; 1 cup cooked cornmeal and raisins, topped with maple syrup; 1/2 cup cottage cheese with pineapple slice; peppermint tea or coffee substitute.

10 am Snack

Two Kiwi fruit, peeled and sliced.

Lunch

Fenugreek tea, 8 oz; large garden salad topped with grated raw zucchini, grated raw beet and finely-ground sunflower seeds; chicken breast without skin, baked with fresh coriander leaves and dill weed; steamed spinach; fresh raspberries and 1/2 cup non-fat natural yogurt.

3 pm Snack

Ak-Mak crackers and 2 oz cheddar cheese.

Dinner

Carrot-celery juice, 8 oz; baked acorn squash, flavored with vegetable broth powder and fine sprinkling of cayenne pepper; Waldorf salad; cooked pearled barley, reheated with peas and pearl onions; 1/2 cup frozen low-fat natural yogurt w/cherry concentrate topping.

Herbal Salad Dressing

1/2 clove garlic	1 tbsp fine chopped basil
1 tbsp chives	1 tbsp chopped parsley
3/4 cup olive oil	1/4 cup wine vinegar

Combine all ingredients in a jar, top and shake; refrigerate for 5 days, shaking the jar now and then.

Day 4, Breakfast

Strawberry-papaya juice, 8 oz; 2 boiled eggs; sliced ripe tomatoes; 2 Ry-Krisp crackers; comfrey-peppermint tea.

10 am Snack

Small-to-medium very ripe banana.

Lunch

Lemon grass tea and apple juice (half and half), 8 oz; small garden salad; salmon steak or fillet (baked or broiled); steamed broccoli; cooked brown rice; slice of melon.

3 pm Snack

Radishes and cucumber slices.

Dinner

Split pea soup, 1 cup; corn-on-the-cob with 1 pat of butter and vegetable broth seasoning; baked sweet potato; Caesar salad; 1/2 cup low-fat yogurt with a handful fresh or frozen blueberries.

GUIDE TO HERBAL SEASONINGS

BEEF: Cloves, cumin, garlic, marjoram, savory, rosemary, bay.
CHEESE: Basil, thyme, sage, oregano, marjoram, fennel, dill.
FISH: Coriander, French tarragon, thyme, parsley, chervil.
FRUIT: Anise, cinnamon, cloves, ginger, mint, sweet cicely.
*LAMB: Garlic, mint, marjoram, rosemary, thyme, oregano.
POULTRY: Savory, sage, fresh coriander leaves, garlic, oregano, rosemary.
SALADS: Basil, chives, garlic, borage, sorrel, burnet, tarragon.
SOUPS: Parsley, rosemary, savory, tarragon, marjoram, bay.
VEGETABLES: Thyme, tarragon, basil, dill, chervil, burnet, marjoram.

*Make slits in the lamb with a sharp knife and stuff herbal seasonings inside.

Day 5, Breakfast

Raspberry-pineapple juice, 8 oz; 1 cup hot, cooked brown rice with raisins, sprinkled with cinnamon and topped with honey or maple syrup; fresh pear.

10 am Snack

Chico-San rice crackers with almond nut butter and 8 oz glass of raw goat's milk.

Lunch

Cup of onion soup; cup of millet; roast leg-of-lamb w/mint jelly; large garden salad topped with shredded raw turnip, raw carrot and raw beet; steamed peas.

3 pm Snack

Feta cheese and Ak-Mak crackers; 1 tsp chlorophyll in glass of water.

Dinner

Barley and kale soup; baked eggplant, steamed Brussels sprouts; steamed parsnips; steamed zucchini; small garden salad; pear slices for dessert.

WATCH FOR CALORIES IN THESE DRESSINGS*

Avocado, 1/3 large	124 calories
Bleu cheese, 2 tbsp	152 calories
French, 2 tbsp	124 calories
Herb, oil and vinegar, 2 tbsp	166 calories
Italian tbsp	166 calories
Lemon juice and oil, 2 tbsp	166 calories
Mayonnaise, 2 tbsp	220 calories
Roquefort, 2 tbsp	152 calories
Thousand island, 2 tbsp	150 calories

*Most can be thinned with non-fat dry milk or buttermilk.

Day 6, Breakfast

Papaya-coconut juice, 8 oz; 1 cup cooked oatmeal; 1/2 cup yogurt with boysenberries; stewed prunes.

10 am Snack

Two celery stalks with sesame butter.

Lunch

Glass of whey, 8 oz; cheese plate with Swiss, cheddar and jack cheese with thin-cut slices of dark rye bread; large garden salad topped with shredded raw zucchini, carrot and beet and sprinkled psyllium husks; sliced fresh peach for dessert.

3 pm Snack

Fresh goat milk (warm, if possible), 8 oz; baked potato; carrot and raisin salad; steamed zucchini, yellow crook-neck squash and cutup tomatoes.

A Word to the Wise

There are many kinds of vegetable and herbal seasonings available in health food stores and even in supermarkets these days, some of which taste salty without containing salt. Break the salt habit and use these instead. Try them all until you find one you like best. Some stores also feature a vegetable broth powder that has a satisfying "salty" flavor. These no-salt seasonings work well on baked potatoes, yams, sweet potatoes, cooked squash, cooked vegetables, boiled or poached eggs, chicken, fish, lamb and beef. A little cayenne pepper may or may not be to your taste, but try it anyway.

Day 7, Breakfast

Pear-apple juice, 8 oz; two poached eggs nested atop large cut cornbread slices; small helping of muesli (add hot water first, then goat's milk later, with a little honey for added sweetness).

10 am Snack

Apple slices, walnuts, celery.

Lunch

Lemon grass tea; broiled trout (with lemon wedges); 3 slices whole wheat French bread (be sparing with the butter); large garden salad with herb-oil-vinegar dressing (no extra toppings); half cup cooked brown rice; pitted dark cherries in yogurt for dessert.

3 pm Snack

Medium ripe banana and a glass of goat's milk.

Dinner

Veal joint broth; 1/2 cup cottage cheese and sliced tomatoes; baked yam; coleslaw; Ak-Mak or Chico-San crackers; bowl of strawberries and fresh pineapple chunks.

I hope you are seeing a pattern in the preceding menus that you can continue to follow on your own, altering to fit your individual taste. If you like to barbecue fish, chicken, lamb and lean beef, go ahead, enjoy yourself. Always remove the skin of the chicken after you barbecue, to reduce the saturated fat intake.

Perhaps the most important point to remember is to keep up with the salad/vegetables/whole grains/fruits and juices parts of the program. If you find your bowel movements increasing to two or more a day, don't be alarmed, that is more normal than once a day or once every two or three days. After your first month on this new food regimen, if you still find that your bowel movements are difficult, sluggish or show other evidence of constipation and underactivity, sprinkle raw psyllium husk (an excellent fiber available at most health food stores) on your salads and vegetables, along with your other seasonings.

If you are not familiar with raw nut and seed butters, they are like peanut butter (unsalted), only milder. You can make them yourself with a Champion Juicer. When freshly made, they are high in vitamin E, fatty acids, calcium and other minerals. A commercially popular brand of sesame seed butter, called tahini, is available at many health food stores. Sometimes other nut and seed butters are available there as well.

SPECIAL HEART DIET—THE LEFT-SIDE DIET

I have encountered individuals with heart problems who did not respond satisfactorily to the low-salt, low-fat regimen previously described, and I will tell you what I did. I changed them to a special heart diet that I call "the left side diet," because the heart is slightly to the left of the midline of the body. I cut out the beef, lamb, fish and chicken and changed them to a diet limited to eggs and milk products as the only animal proteins. I also increased the amount of starches to make up for the elimination of the fish, chicken and so forth. The high proportions of vegetables remained the same.

WHAT DO I MEAN BY STARCHES?

All fruits, vegetables and whole grains are considered carbohydrates, but the vegetables and grains with the most simple carbohydrate content are often called starches. These include, but are not limited to, buckwheat, brown rice, oats, rye, millet, yellow cornmeal, sweet potatoes, yams, potatoes, lentils and barley. Whole barley can't be eaten, no matter how long you cook it, because the husks are too tough. So, we use pearled or "hulled" barley, in this case.

On a high-starch regimen, the individuals I referred to in the beginning showed great improvement, as revealed through blood pressure changes and blood cholesterol and triglyceride levels. They also felt better, which is nice, but not conclusive, as cardiovascular problems go.

NUTRITION FOR THE HEART

We find that nutritionists today are often in the position where they need to evaluate an organ disturbance or disease to determine what chemical elements are missing in the body. Every disease or disturbance is associated with chemical deficiencies. There is no organ that lacks just one chemical element. Whenever there is a sickness, every organ in the body needs many different elements in order to keep the various structures alive that exist within that organ.

Most organs have muscle structure and they have a ligament structure. They have a tendon structure, nerves, blood vessels and lymph vessels all with their own activity. The muscle tissues need a good deal of potassium, but all tendons, ligaments, nerves and all the blood and lymph vessels need silicon and calcium. Also, of all things, they need sodium to make the blood vessels elastic and movable, active and pliable so the walls can expand and contract. The heart arteries must be strong to contain the rhythmic pressure changes of the blood as it is pumped by the heart.

The heart has muscle tissue to drive the heartbeat, connective tissue to hold it together, membranes around the heart muscle (and lining its chambers) and this is all very tough, pliable material. This roughness comes through the chemical elements calcium, silicon and sodium.

These elements contribute to the proper activity of the whole heart and while the heart is primarily a muscle organ, we cannot think that only the muscle is depleted in all heart conditions. All the various tissues that make up the heart have to be fed, and there are more chemical elements needed to do this.

While the heart is strong, we cannot have even one weakness there or the heart may break down from that weakness.

IT ISN'T ENOUGH TO EAT THE RIGHT FOODS

Although we must eat the right foods to get the chemical elements the heart needs, it is very important to make sure that the digestion is good. Unless we digest and assimilate our foods, we don't get the elements we need. Many people don't realize that good digestion requires sodium in the walls of the stomach and small intestine. Now, they are taking sodium away in heart troubles today. This is because people use too much salt, and table salt doesn't have the right kind of sodium for the heart. They say some people use 20 or 30 grams of salt per day, and that is far too much for the heart and arteries. This is pure, refined inorganic chemical salt, not food salt. We only need about one gram of sodium per day and this is provided naturally, by our foods.

I strongly recommend that you switch to one of the popular and taste-pleasing herb-and-vegetable seasonings as a substitute for salt. If you must use salt, change to sea salt and use it sparingly.

I call sodium the "youth element" because it keeps tissue pliable, young and supple. This organic sodium that we are discussing is needed by structures of the heart other than the muscle structure. The muscle structure needs potassium, but the rest of the heart, such as the valves, tendons, connective tissue and membranes need sodium for flexibility.

WE MUST FEED THE WHOLE BODY

We have to consider that we're breaking down the heart mainly because of conditions in the other organs in the body, sluggishness in the veins, a slowed-down metabolism and poor circulation from our lack of exercise. The legs are pumps that move the venous blood back to the heart, but if we are not using those legs, the blood doesn't move as it should. We also need the right nutrition to keep the artery and vein walls strong and flexible.

So, we have to work toward a nutritionally-balanced body. Potassium takes care of a good deal of the acids in the muscles, and sodium takes care of acids in the joints and digestive system. The right balance between sodium and potassium helps to regulate the pH of the blood and the amount of water in the body. Sodium and potassium are needed in the transfer of nutrients across cell membranes and in the passage of electrical impulses through the nerves. Sodium and potassium are two of the most important and widely-used food elements in the whole body.

When we stop and think now that the heart is the strongest organ in the body, yet often lacking in certain chemical elements that it needs to work right and to prevent breakdowns, it makes sense to have a list of those foods that are good for the heart. We find that there are a few recipes that we should have so we can make "heart meals." We must have a good starch every day for the heart activity, and I mean a whole starch, such as brown rice or a baked potato. Also we have to have a certain amount of sodium, and we can look to the green vegetables for some of the sodium we need in our body. All salad vegetables contain sodium and so do homemade soups.

Both soups and salads are rich in the natural chemical elements needed to build a whole body.

We are finding out that we need a certain amount of fluorine foods along with the calcium in our diet. Fluorine only comes in raw foods. I recommend raw goat milk, raw cheese, liquid whey and possibly a little raw quince. Calcium fluoride is found in nature. Fluorine is destroyed by heat in cooking or even in pasteurization. Fluorine is a very unstable element, but it comes in raw milk products and should be considered as one of the chemical elements that strengthen the heart.

We need a certain amount of oxygen in the body and we get this from the air we breathe. Without iron in the blood, we cannot attract the oxygen from the air in our lungs. We can also increase our oxygen intake by regular exercise.

WALK—FOR YOUR HEART'S SAKE

People with heart troubles are nearly always told by their doctors to walk half an hour every morning. Why? To improve circulation, strengthen the heart, get the oxygen from fresh air, improve muscle tone, help bring about better bowel activity, cheer up the mind and start the day off right. Walking is a very wonderful thing for the legs and so is a certain amount of swimming. These exercises help the heart and circulation.

Dr. Paul Dudley White, the heart doctor I admire most, took care of President Dwight Eisenhower after his heart attack. He made the president walk—every day. Dr. White said, "The legs are the pumps that bring the venous blood back to the heart." Very few people realize how the blood slows down after it reaches the extremities of the body—head, hands and feet—and begins its return journey to the heart through the venous system. They used to talk about "tired blood." Venous blood has the oxygen used up, and it is loaded with carbonic acid, carbon dioxide and metabolic wastes. People who sit a lot or have limited movement on their jobs need to learn ways to get that venous blood back to the heart.

Foot baths are very good for the circulation, hot and cold foot baths. We find manipulation, massage and acupuncture, chiropractic, osteopathy and Shiatzu, all of these can help the circulation and keep the proper nerve supply open to the heart and to the arterial system throughout the whole body. There's no use working with just the heart when the rest of the body is dragging down the heart activity.

Vitamin E helps to bring oxygen to the tissues, so it is very necessary in most heart troubles. We get it from raw nuts and seeds and whole grains. We find that the B vitamins are necessary in most heart troubles, and these are found most in meat, chicken and fish, as well as dairy products. The best vegetable source of vitamin B-12 is chlorella, in alga found in health food stores. Chlorella is very high in chlorophyll, nature's best cleanser, and it is also high in DNA and RNA, the nucleic acids. These are needed to help rebuild damaged tissue. The brain needs the B-vitamins. The brain is very important in heart health.

THE IMPORTANCE OF BRAIN NUTRITION

You can't have a healthy, nicely-working heart without a healthy, nicely-working brain. The brain controls the oxygen supply, the blood pH, the metabolic rate, the glandular secretions, the amount of water in the body and influences the heart rate and blood pressure. If we want to have a healthy heart, we must take care of the brain.

The brain needs silicon, sulfur, phosphorus, lecithin, cholesterol and vitamin B-Complex. The medulla is often called "the chest brain." It is the dynamo for keeping the heart beating properly.

I am positive that no one has heart trouble without having trouble in the medulla. Vitamin B and lecithin are the two most important things we have to consider in this case, and lecithin is also a great dissolver of cholesterol and should be used along with sodium to keep up the circulation well and to keep youthfulness throughout the whole body so that overworking of the heart doesn't take place.

One last thought in this chapter is that we should keep away from vitality wasters. When recuperating from a heart attack or trying to prevent heart trouble, we should consider avoiding activities that waste our time and energy. Avoid tasks and people that drag you down and never build you up. Watch your attitude—worry is a vitality waster. Take time to smell the roses and admire the stars, but stay away from nagging, complaining, whining, negative, depressing or spiteful people.

A good heart-building attitude is to look for the best in life and people, and leave the rest. Be good to yourself, and you'll feel more like being good to others.

HIGHEST SODIUM FOODS

Veal joint broth and powdered whey (cow's milk or goat milk) are highly-concentrated sources of sodium. Goat milk or whey and black mission figs are the superior sodium combination (and this is also a champion arthritis remedy).

High sodium foods include:

Apples	Kale
Apricots, dried	Kelp
Asparagus	Lentils
Barley	Milk, raw
Beets and greens	Mustard greens
Cabbage, red	Okra
Carrots	Olives, black
Celery	Parsley
Cheese	Peas, dried
Chickpeas, dried	Peppers, hot, red, dried
Coconut	Prunes
Collard greens	Raisins
Dandelion greens	Sesame seeds
Dates	Spinach, New Zealand

Dulse
Egg yolks
Figs
Fish
Goat milk, raw
Horseradish

Strawberries
Sunflower seeds
Swiss chard
Turnips
Veal joint broth
Whey

Fair sources of sodium include other cabbage, water chestnuts, garlic, peaches (dried), radishes, broccoli, Brussels sprouts, cashews and a dried goat whey called Capri Mineral Whey, available from Mt. Capra Cheese, 279 S.W. 9th Street, Chehalis, WA 98532.

HIGHEST POTASSIUM FOODS

Sun-dried black olives and potato peeling broth are two of the best sources of potassium. Dulse, kelp and Irish moss are also good. Other high potassium foods are listed below. Remember that excessive heat destroys potassium, as does food processing.

Almonds
Anise seeds
Apples
Apple cider vinegar
Apple peelings
Apricots, dried
Bananas
Beans, dried red, pinto,
 white, mung, string
Beets (red, yellow)
Beet greens
Black cherries
Blueberries
Broccoli
Brussels sprouts
Carrots

Escarole
Figs, dried
Fish
Goat milk
Grapes
Green turtle
Jerusalem artichoke
Kale
Kelp
Leaf lettuce
Lentils
Lima beans, dried
Olives
Parsley
Parsnips
Peaches, bitter

Cashews	Pears, dried
Cheese, brown	Pecans
Cucumbers	Potato peelings
Currants	Raisins
Dates	Rice bran
Dulse	Rice polishings
Egg white	Sage tea
Sesame seeds, whole	Tomatoes (red, yellow)
Soy milk	Turnips
Soybeans, dried	Walnuts
Spinach	Watercress
Sunflower seeds	Wheat bran
Swiss chard	Wheat germ

TABLE OF FOODS CONTAINING HEART SALTS

Nature prepares heart salts, if we only provide the foods they are in. Heart salts are found in the foods in the following list.

Figs (black, fresh)	Leaf lettuce
Rice bran muffins	Endive
Ripe, sun-dried olives	Chinese cabbage
Rye-meal bread	Steamed spinach
Veal joint jelly	Cherries
Beets	Broth from fresh bones
Nettle salad	Sun-dried prunes
Celery	Goat milk cottage cheese
Egg whites	Dill
Green figs	Crab broth
Lobster broth	Fresh crabs
Lobsters	Oysters
Lamb chops	Swiss chard
Roquefort cheese	Smoked halibut
Egg yolk/orange juice shake	Parsley
Fresh strawberries	Sole
Smelt	Chervil
Broccoli	Turnip leaves
Oyster broth	

CHAPTER 11

SUPPLEMENTS FOR A HEALTHY HEART

We must recognize, right at the start, that taking supplements such as one-a-day, ultra-vitamin-mineral tablets cannot possibly compensate for imbalanced food habits and a high heart risk lifestyle. If you smoke cigarettes, there is no vitamin supplement that can protect your lungs and cardiovascular system from damage. If you refuse to exercise for at least a half hour every day, no amount of vitamin E can make up for that lack of exercise.

The point is, supplements only work well when you are already on the road with a right-living program and an appropriate diet, such as we have discussed in the previous chapters.

Now here are some supplements I can recommend to help protect your cardiovascular system from future problems and to help reverse already existing conditions. They will help only if you are making a significant effort to follow most of the lifestyle guidelines in this book.

Alfalfa Tablets. Alfalfa is high in iron to help oxygenate the blood and high in chlorophyll, nature's best cleansing agent, a good blood builder. Alfalfa tablets should be cracked before swallowing, and taken with meals, eight at each mealtime. The fiber and chlorophyll in alfalfa tablets are excellent for improving bowel tone and regularity and for feeding the friendly bowel flora.

Beta Carotene. Also known as pro-vitamin A, cuts heart attack risk. Findings from the Nurses' Health Study showed that women eating a cup per day of beta carotene foods had 40% fewer strokes and 22% fewer heart attacks than those only having 1/4 cup or less.

Chlorophyll. Liquid chlorophyll is available in most health food stores. Take 1 teaspoon chlorophyll in a glass of water three times daily for cleansing and building the blood. Chlorophyll is rich in iron and magnesium, iron to build the blood, magnesium to detoxify metabolic acids in the heart. The chlorophyll molecule is the same structure as the hemoglobin molecule in the blood, except it has a magnesium atom at the center instead of iron.

Honey. Raw, unpasteurized honey is a wonderful food for the heart. It is a clean, natural source of food energy.

Honeybee Pollen. Analysts say this is the most complete food known, containing all necessary amino acids, many enzymes, oils, vitamins, minerals and natural sugars. It has been used to raise the red blood cell count and lower high blood pressure.

Propolis. This substance is made of resin gathered by bees from buds of trees. It is 5% pollen, 30% wax, 55% resins and balms and 10% oils. It contains many vitamins, minerals and flavonoids. Studies in the USSR show that it helps hypertension and vascular problems. Studies in China indicate that it lowers blood triglycerides.

Ginseng. Tienchi ginseng is reported to provide relief from the pain of angina pectoris. Used over a period of several months, it may help normalize blood pressure. Ginseng, in general, is considered a tonic for promoting long life and healthy sexuality.

Wheat Germ or Wheat Germ Oil. A tablespoon of wheat germ twice a day or a teaspoon of wheat germ oil twice a day is an excellent way to make sure the body is getting all the natural vitamin E it needs. Vitamin E increases the oxygenation of the blood, which directly benefits the heart.

Evening Primrose Oil. European studies report that use of evening primrose oil lowers high blood pressure, lowers the blood level of cholesterol and helps prevent thrombosis.

Dried Goat Whey (made by Mt. Capra Cheese, 279 S.W. 9th Street, Chehalis, WA 96532). This is the richest source of bio-organic potassium I know, and is also a nice source of food sodium. The heart is a potassium organ which needs a modest amount of bio-organic sodium to nourish its membranes, ligaments and tendons. Potassium is used in the heart muscle to neutralize metabolic acid wastes to prevent them from having healthy cells as they pass into the lymphatic system.

Hawthorne Berry Tea. This herbal tea is considered perhaps the most helpful heart support herbal remedy, especially for the elderly. It may be used together with capsicum to aid circulation.

Lecithin. Soy lecithin granules can be purchased in a health food store. Raw nuts and seeds are rich in lecithin, but cooking destroys it. Lecithin is not only needed to help keep cholesterol in soluble form in the bloodstream, but to feed and support the brain centers (such as the medulla) that regulate heart and vascular activity. Some studies indicate that lecithin may help reverse arteriosclerosis, used along with a proper diet and exercise program.

Sesame Seeds. Sesame seeds are high in vitamin E, calcium and oils needed for glandular support. The Turks use halvah and tahini, and they are among the strongest people in the world. Sesame seeds should be ground finely or made into a seed butter or seed milk drink. Tahini can be found in many health food stores.

Rice Bran Syrup (or rice polishings). Rich in B-Complex vitamins, rice bran syrup provides energy; promotes the metabolism of carbohydrates, fats and proteins; and supports the nervous system.

Niacin. Otherwise known as vitamin B-3, niacin causes a flush to the head and shoulders, driving the blood circulation. Nutritionists have used up to a gram of niacin after each meal to lower blood cholesterol and reduce the risk of heart attack.

Catalyn. This is the brand name of a wonderful B vitamin put out by Standard Process Laboratories, which I have recommended for many years to patients with heart trouble.

Vitamin E. Women taking 100 milligrams of vitamin E daily had 36% fewer heart attacks than those taking 30 milligrams or less. The women used supplements, but foods with vitamin E would work as well or better. Whole grains, raw nuts and seeds, green vegetables, wheat germ and wheat germ oil are natural sources of vitamin E. One teaspoon of liquid chlorophyll in a glass of water is good for the heart.

Veal Joint Broth. This provides food sodium for the digestive system, joints and non-muscle heart tissues, as an alternative to table salt, which I regard as dangerous. Buy a fresh, uncut veal joint, wash, cover half with water in a large cooking pot and add: 2 cups potato peelings, 1/2 cup okra and 1 teaspoon powdered okra, 1 stalk chopped celery, 1 parsnip, 1 onion, 2 grated beets, 1/2 cup parsley. Simmer 4-5 hours, strain off solids and drink the broth. Store the rest in the refrigerator.

Potassium Broth. Peel 1 potatoes 1/4 inch deep, simmer these in 3 cups of water for 15 minutes; strain and drink broth.

Hawthorne Berry Tea. This tea is an excellent tonic for the heart. You may use one teaspoon of honey in it two to three times a day.

Chlorella. This single-celled edible alga is growing in popularity as people discover its health-support benefits. It is the highest known natural source of chlorophyll (1.7%), and has been used to lower high blood pressure in Japanese research studies. It also lowered cholesterol and triglyceride levels in a 3-month study of 16 patients at the Wakahisa Hospital.

Seven-Day Tissue Cleansing. Using a 7-day combination of nutritional supplements and 2 colemas daily for that time (a colema is similar to a high enema), I have seen triglyceride readings as high as 1403 mg/dl drop to 325 mg/dl. Other patients with high blood cholesterol or weakness due to aftereffects of stroke or heart attack reported excellent improvement. The 7-day tissue cleansing program is fully described in my book *Tissue Cleansing Through Bowel Management.*

Heart Protomorphagen. Protomorphagens are usually desiccated, powdered organs from cattle, used to provide nutrients nearly the same as those required in comparable human organs. I have seen many patients helped by taking heart protomorphagens along with a good diet.

WHAT DO I DO NEXT?

You can't use all the supplements or procedures I have just described, but you can use some and experiment with others described here. They are all foods and safe to use.

My personal recommendation is that you begin by using a liquid chlorophyll drink 3 times a day, a teaspoon of honeybee pollen 2 times a day (after meals), wheat germ, dried goat whey, rice bran syrup and polishings and potassium broth (once or twice a week).

I highly recommend that you read my book *Tissue Cleansing Through Bowel Management* to understand the role of the elimination organs, especially the bowel, in health and disease.

If you follow a regular exercise program, make the lifestyle changes I have recommended, adopt a Healthy Heart Food Regimen and use the supplements carefully. I believe you will be feeling wonderful in a year or less. Why a year or less? Because I tell my patients it takes a year for old tissue to be replaced by new tissue. In a year or so, you can have a completely new heart. Isn't that wonderful?

CHAPTER 12

55 WAYS TO PREVENT HEART DISEASE AND BUILD A HEALTHY HEART

1. Don't smoke.
2. Reduce salt to less than 2 gm/day.
3. Eliminate or reduce red meat in your diet.
4. Use more poultry and fish in place of red meat.
5. Change from cow's milk to raw seed milk and nut milk drinks, and raw seed and nut butters.
6. Do not overeat or snake between meals.
7. If you are overweight for your height and bone structure, reduce to your right weight.
8. Restrict the percentage of fat calories to 30% of total calories in daily diet.
9. Lower your blood cholesterol to less than 180 mg/dl.
10. Eliminate from your diet fried foods, foods cooked in fat and foods containing oils baked at over 212 degrees F.
11. Minimize the use of refined, processed, packaged and otherwise unnaturally altered foods.
12. Include enough high-fiber vegetables, fruits and whole vegetables, fruits and whole grains in your diet to have regular bowel movements after each meal.
13. Use vitamin E-rich foods and foods high in lecithin to reduce clotting tendency of blood, oxygenate tissues and help prevent cholesterol deposits in the arteries.

14. Minimize the use of refined white sugar, high-sugar-containing soft drinks and all foods containing a high concentration of sugar. (High sugar intake increases blood cholesterol.)
15. Avoid using alcohol to excess.
16. Eliminate gassy foods from your diet.
17. Avoid commercial "health" products such as antacid aids for indigestion and other products high in inorganic sodium salts.
18. Use plenty of high-potassium foods such as whey, bananas, olives, potatoes, parsley, blueberries, watercress, green peppers, peaches, figs and all vegetables.
19. Avoid potassium-leaching foods and drinks such as sugar, alcohol and caffeinated drinks.
20. Avoid low blood sugar, which stresses the adrenal glands and causes loss of potassium.
21. Use chlorella tablets, liquid chlorophyll and acidophilus to keep the bowel clean and in proper balance of flora.
22. Use psyllium husks, oat bran, rice bran or wheat bran to prevent or get rid of constipation.
23. Take good care of the bowel—keep it regular, clean and free of excess gas.
24. Get at least half an hour of vigorous, aerobic exercise before breakfast (if possible) to increase oxygenation of the blood, strengthen the heart and increase the metabolic rate. Work up to exercise **slowly**, day by day. Exercise to music.
25. Avoid strenuous exercise or physical labor when not accustomed to it.
26. If your job is physically demanding, take **real rest breaks** mid-morning and afternoon, not just "coffee breaks."
27. Get 8 hours of uninterrupted sleep every night.
28. Avoid or control stress in your life by learning relaxation techniques such as deep breathing exercises, visualizations of calm, beautiful scenes and positive affirmations.

29. If you work at "Ulcers, Inc.," it is time to change jobs for your health's sake.
30. Don't take your work home with you, physically or mentally.
31. Do yourself a big health favor—love your spouse and show it often. Express affection regularly with words, gifts, touches, hugs, appreciation, thankfulness, smiles and love notes.
32. Spend enough time with your children to feel good about being a parent. Play with them, listen to them, love them.
33. Avoid being overscheduled, overworked, overwhelmed, overtired, overemotional, overhurried or over anything.
34. Work out financial problems by putting plans and schedules on paper, **getting them off your mind and keeping them off your mind.**
35. When you go on vacation, make it a real vacation: rest, relax and enjoy.
36. Obey the Golden Rule: Do unto others as you would have them do unto you.
37. Learn to forgive and forget.
38. Learn to let go of emotions that disturb the heart—hate, anger, unforgiveness, bitterness, resentment, jealousy, envy and others.
39. Learn to lower your blood pressure, if it is too high, through relaxation training.
40. Vitamin supplements that may help lower blood cholesterol are B-Complex, niacin, C, D, E, F. Niacin has been shown to reduce liver production of cholesterol.
41. Make sure you are using a balanced food regimen to nourish your whole body, so that every organ, gland and tissue supports the heart and does not drag on it.
42. Use skin brushing in the morning and evening to increase elimination from the skin.
43. Drink 3 glasses of water upon rising in the morning to cleanse the kidneys.

44. Take barefoot walks in the grass or sand early each morning to improve circulation. Start out easy.

45. Use Kneipp baths to increase circulation to legs and head.

46. Hawthorne berry tea helps oxygenate the blood and heart.

47. Have a hobby that relaxes your mind and takes your attention away from troubles.

48. Use a slanting board to get better circulation to the brain and relief from prolapsus pressure. Be careful.

49. Colema treatments can reduce blood cholesterol and triglycerides dramatically in only 7 days, if the program in my book *Tissue Cleansing Through Bowel Management* is properly followed.

50. Eliminate anemia by using blackberry juice, black cherry juice, chlorella tablets (10 each meal), chlorophyll-rich foods and bee pollen.

51. Ginseng acts as a tonic to reduce the effects of stress on the mind, heart and blood pressure.

52. Heart protomorphagen may be used to ensure the availability of all nutrients needed for building and maintaining a healthy heart.

53. Take a walk. It is one of the best exercises known to prevent cardiovascular disease.

54. Get a complete physical exam from your doctor, including an electrocardiogram, to check your health, in general, and your heart's health, in particular. Talk to your doctor about heart health and your lifestyle, especially your diet and exercise.

55. Chiropractic treatments can often relieve tensions around the heart.

CHAPTER 13

HEART ZONE ANALYSIS

There are two great misunderstandings made concerning the development, diagnosis and proper treatment of heart diseases and various problems of the heart. First, the relation of the heart (or any other organ) to the whole body is seldom considered. Second, the role of constitutional weaknesses in the development of a disease is often ignored or overlooked. We may consider what this means by having a look at how a human embryo develops.

In the formation of the embryo, the first organized structure to develop is the gut tube, which later becomes the gastrointestinal system. Soon after this tiny, elementary organ appears, microscopic "buds" begin to appear along the gut tube. These "buds" are collections of cells that will become the vital organs of the growing fetus.

One of these buds becomes the heart. This heart emerges from gut tube and is surrounded by gut tissue. This surface membrane is called the pericardium. Wherever there is a constitutional weakness in the gut tube at the site where the heart bud emerges, that weakness will continue to exist throughout life. (This is true of all organs that emerge from the primitive gut tube.) Constitutional weakness in any organ indicates a greater vulnerability to dysfunction and disease than we find in normal organs.

We must learn to view the body as a community of organs, glands, tissues and processes that are interdependent in the work they do and in the condition of the specialized cells they are made of. A weak organ is different from a normal-to-strong organ in its relation to the whole body and to other organs. Its needs are greater and its contributions are smaller. Stronger organs may have to work harder to make up for the shortcomings of weaker organs.

For these reasons, I believe most heart trouble is a secondary condition. There are risk factors and contributing factors, but they would seldom be able to do as much harm to a constitutional weakness. There are many things that contribute to heart trouble. But, if we would begin to deal with heart problems by taking care of and strengthening the whole body, I don't believe we would have so many persons disabled and dying from heart problems.

When I encounter a patient with heart trouble, I look at the overall situation. I consider the constitutional weakness as it has come down through the family. I look at the reflex relationship between the heart and the bowel as it originated in the embryo. I estimate the effects upon the heart of the four elimination channels, which are nearly always underactive in heart patients. The constitutionally weak heart, in my experience, can only take so much strain, stress, nutritional deficiencies and exposure to metabolic acid wastes. To reverse the pathway of heart disease requires a careful remodelling of the patient's lifestyle, attitudes and personal priorities. The patient's nutrition and exercise profiles must be carefully evaluated and changed as necessary. We may consider tissue cleansing methods to hasten detoxification and quicken bowel transit time. All of this requires some means of assessing whether our program is doing the patient any good.

To identify and monitor heart conditions, related body processes and the effectiveness of treatment methods, I have found the science of Iridology most helpful. Computerized iris analysis has proven to be a valid and reliable tool in my work in the detection of heart disease. It may take another 10 years for people to understand and appreciate iridology, but I predict its widespread acceptance in the future for the management of cardiac conditions.

With the preceding introduction, I would like to present the following article, which I wrote nearly five years ago for the magazine <u>Iridologists International and the Allied Healing Arts</u>, Vol. VI, Issue 1, 1991.

Some of the nice things that can come from the use of the computer are the topographical maps that it can make. Some are in color and some are in black and white. From these, we can see the qualities of tissue ranging from acute to chronic and degenerative. This information can be of tremendous value when determining the condition of the heart.

ANALYSIS OF HEART ZONE (LS)

Dr. Jensen's Observations. Here, we have a photograph of the iris. A lacuna can be seen at exactly 3 o'clock, which

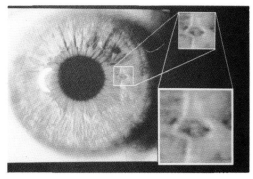

Iris photo of left eye showing lacuna in heart section.

is the heart zone. There seems to be a separation within the autonomic nerve wreath showing an inherent weakness. Toxic material has settled in the inherent weakness and the reflex condition is working in the bowel region as well as on the opposite side of the heart zone in the bronchial tube structure.

In this situation, the heart is "between a rock and a hard place." The bowel is the beginning of the reflex condition. The bronchial tube is also involved in the reflex condition. The heart is located directly between the bowel and the bronchial tubes.

The photograph below shows this heart lesion by a topographical map in various colors and depths. The bar displays colors ranging from acute to degenerate. From the map, we can see that the chronic and degenerate areas are located throughout the heart section (see enlarged view). Also notice that the top fibers are white, indicating an acute stage of inflammation. Deeper fibers are very dark in color and show degenerate tissue, or an extreme chronic condition existing in this particular organ. This represents toxic settlement, inflammation, mineral deficiency, overacidity, underactivity and lack of blood.

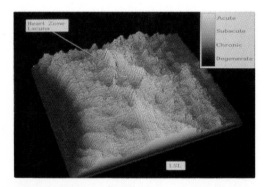

Perspective topographic surface plot with gray-scale elevation (brightness) contour bands for heart zone area.

In the figure below, we have the gray scale elevation and the contour bands for the heart zone. It is the same area as shown in Figure 2 (above). With the gray scale, we can better see the topography (indentations and elevations) of the fiber structures as they are found deep within the iris. This is a good in-depth study for the examiner of the iris.

As shown on the bar, white represents an acute condition and the darker colors represent deeper and deeper levels of degeneration, with black as the most chronic.

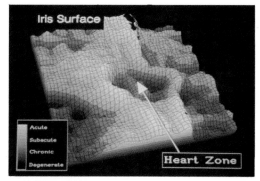

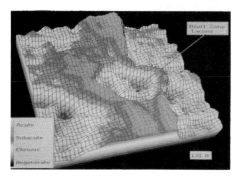

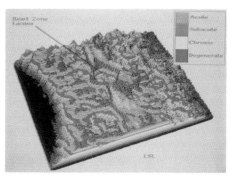

These 3 photos show perspective topographic surface plot with gray-scale (TOP and in color MID and BOTTOM) elevation (brightness) contour bands for heart zone area.

ANALYSIS OF HEART ZONE (AZ)

Dr. Jensen's Observations. Notice the marking for the heart area and the wreath that goes around it. See how the bronchial tube is on the outside marked bronchial and a marking coming from the bowel above it. It begins there because the constitutional makeup of the bowel is always weaker than any other tissue in the body. However, all inherent weaknesses are found in constitutional weaknesses in the body which are represented in the iris by the closeness of the fibers or the separation of them.

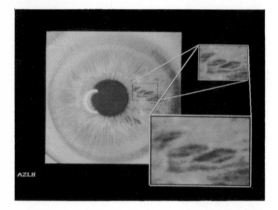

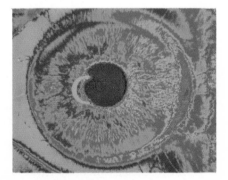

TOP: Iris photo with enlargement of heart zone area.
BOTTOM: Pseudocolor mapping of iris image shown above.

The figure below is a definite heart case. This person has had a couple of heart attacks. We are dealing with a history of heart troubles. This is not a theory but a very definite demonstration. The condition in the heart area usually shows up as a trapezoid when the wreath is separated. The heart is part of the nervous system or a part of the autonomic nerve wreath. The medulla that keeps the heart beating and giving it its normal rhythm is part of the brain and nervous system and transferred through the autonomic nervous system to the heart region.

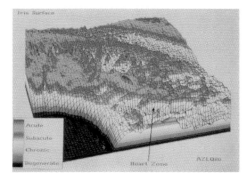

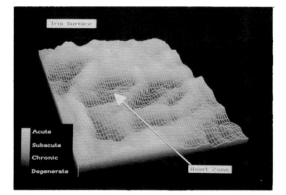

TOP: *Perspective topographic surface plot with color-coded elevation (brightness) contour bands for upper right quadrant of iris.* BOTTOM: *Perspective topographic surface plot with gray-scale elevation (brightness) contour bands for heart zone area.*

ANALYSIS OF HEART ZONE (GM)

Dr. Jensen's Observations. Always look for a definite heart lesion when a person has a heart disturbance. There are also other problems that contribute to the heart trouble itself. In the case of my patient, the greatest thing that is shown here is the arcus senilis, which is in the brain area. Because of the arcus senilis and poor circulation, there is not enough blood going to the medulla, which regulates the heart rhythm.

The adrenal gland, as shown, is underactive. Without adrenal function, the heart does not have the necessary stimulation to pump as it should. So, this patient was a prime candidate for a heart attack because of the contributing factors involved. I told him about this heart condition, and a couple of months later, he had a heart attack.

The science of Iridology looks to the whole body through the iris because it recognizes that all of the parts work together. There is a unity in disease; there is a unity in health. We cannot just treat one symptom. We must take care of the whole body. We must assist all of the inherent weaknesses in order to strengthen the whole. We must cleanse the toxic materials that are settled in these inherent weaknesses and nourish them with the proper nutrients to make them well and strong.

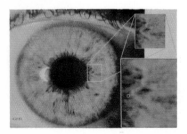 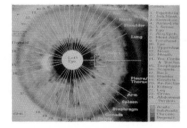

The whole lifestyle of my friend had to be changed. If he was living in stress or fear, he was destroying the adrenal glands which leads to heart troubles.

The white ring around the iris is indicative of a cholesterol ring and hardening of the arteries. This was just discovered by the American Optometric Association a year ago (at the time of this writing), however, I have had this information in my books for over 20 years. There are nerve rings in this patient indicating stress. Stress taxes the heart directly. So with lifestyle education, we can often prevent disease, heart disease and heart attacks. With lifestyle change, positive thinking, tissue cleansing and good nutrition, we can heal from within out.

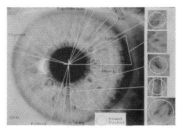

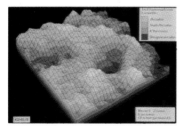

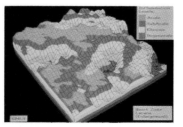

*Iris photo with enlargements of bowel pockets and heart zone lacuna.
mid: Perspective topographic surface plot with (TOP) gray-scaled (MID AND
BOTTOM) color elevation (brightness) contour bands for heart zone area.*

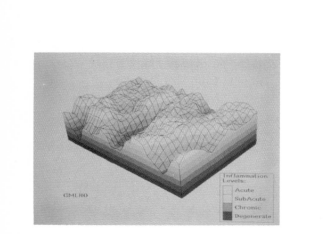

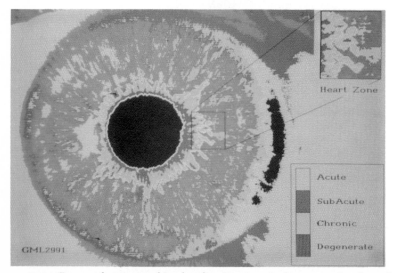

TOP: Gray-scale topographic plot showing a vertical cross section through the heart zone lacuna. BOTTOM: Four-level pseudocolor contour map showing inflammation levels, with enlargement of heart zone.

ANALYSIS OF HEART ZONE (WE)

Dr. Jensen's Observations. This is a heart case of a person with Marfan's syndrome. This is a hereditary condition that affects the connective tissue, bones, muscles, ligaments and skeletal structures. These people are tall and lanky with long arms, fingers and legs. They lack calcium and are typically affected with heart trouble.

As we look to the heart area, we see that it is the blackest and the darkest in the entire iris. It is within the autonomic nerve wreath. On one side of the heart, the bronchial tubes are not well and on the other side of the heart, the bowel is showing a toxic material forming the beginning of a reflex condition which can, over time, wear down and weaken the heart itself.

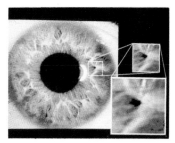

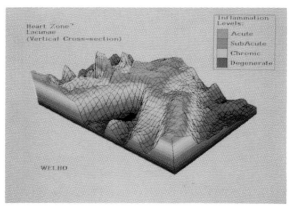

This shows a perspective topographic surface plot with color-coded elevation (brightness) contour bands for heart zone area.

We should note also that this man died of heart trouble. He was a definite heart case, as well as a case of Marfan's syndrome.

We find in Marfan's syndrome that the ligaments and tendons are weak and the heart is made up of muscle tissue which is also weak in a person with this disease. They lack calcium. In this person, you can see that the spine, which is a calcium organ, is in need of calcium. It doesn't have the support from a nutritional standpoint that it should.

We are seeking markings in people of like conditions that would show up the same in the irides.

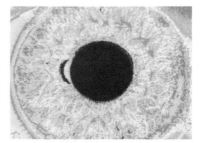

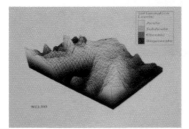

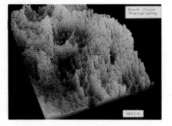

TOP: Pseudocolor mapping of iris image. MID: Perspective topographic surface plat w/gray-scale elevation for heart zone. BOTTOM: Gray-scale topographic map of spine area in left iris.

WARNING
TO PEOPLE WHO WANT TO AVOID
HEART TROUBLE

It is hard to warn a person concerning the risk of heart trouble in the future, but heart trouble can be prevented or greatly reduced by taking the proper measures. During World War I, Denmark was forced to reduce its intake of meat and dairy products. Under the direction of a physician, Dr. Hindhede, 80% of the hogs and 34% of the cattle were slaughtered. The national diet changed to predominantly whole grains, vegetables, fruit and limited dairy products. Their whole grain bread was enriched with extra bran. As a result, the death rate dropped by 17%, the lowest in Europe. Unfortunately, the Danes went back to their high-fat, high-heart-risk diet after the war.

I feel one of the greatest problems in the USA today is a diet and food habits that bring on heart disease. In the U.S. today, 52% of the people are overweight and many people use excessive amounts of table salt. The sodium in the salt attracts water. This can be responsible for extra weight in the body. Table salt is processed at high heat and reacts in the body to cause side effects that contribute to hardening of the arteries and high blood pressure. The good news is that we can control our diets and salt intake. The bad news is that most people don't.

I went to the Hunza Valley of Pakistan 30 years ago. This is the little valley in the Himalayas that had no diseases whatsoever—no cancer, no hospitals, no doctors and no drugstores. However, just after I left, a Japanese expedition visited the Hunza Valley, and found that the people were short of iodine, which is needed by the thyroid gland that controls the metabolism. They found goiters but then never found an overweight Hunzacut. They lived very long lives. I found men there who were 110 to 140 years of age. There was no heart disease among them.

Salt has an effect in the body that is signaled by a sodium ring around the iris, as we have noted for many years in our work with Iridology. I have often encountered the sodium ring in the eyes of overweight persons and in persons who worked on ships, such as sailors. The classic case of health problems among sailors is told in the story of the German cruiser "Kronprinz Wilhelm" during World War I. The crew of this cruiser lived for over 8 months on food taken from British and French merchant vessels before the ships were evacuated and sunk. This German crew became so sick they had to come into the U.S. port for treatment. Naval ship crews often had diets rich in salted meat and fish in days past, low in fresh fruit, vegetables and whole grain foods. Dietary deficiencies, together with heavy salting of preserved foods, were and are very dangerous to the heart.

MENU OF THE GERMAN KRONPRINZ WILHELM

Alfred McCann gives the menu of the German sailors aboard the Wilhelm. We find that he has the following to say about the diet and illnesses, according to his book, *Science of Eating*.

"From the ship's cook, with the chief surgeon's assistance, I obtained the following chart, showing just what the meals consisted of, prior to the breaking out of the disease described by scientific men as 'beri-beri.' The chart...tells just what was behind the beri-beri, acidosis, neuritis, jail edema, trench edema, war nephritis, pellagra, or whatever term is adopted to describe the sufferings of the men."

Monday. Breakfast: Cheese, oatmeal, condensed milk, white bread, butter (oleo), coffee, sugar. Dinner: Pea soup, canned vegetables served in juice that stood in cans, roast beef, boiled potatoes, white bread, coffee, condensed milk, sugar.

Tuesday. Breakfast: Sausage, white bread, butter (oleo), fried potatoes, coffee, condensed milk, sugar. Dinner: Potato soup, canned vegetables served in juice that stood in cans, pot roast of beef, boiled potatoes, white bread, butter (oleo), coffee, condensed milk, sugar.

Wednesday. Breakfast: Corned beef, white bread, butter (oleo), fried potatoes, coffee, condensed milk, sugar. Dinner: Beef soup, roast beef, boiled potatoes, white bread, butter (oleo), coffee, condensed milk, sugar.

Thursday. Breakfast: Smoked ham, cheese, white bread, butter (oleo), condensed milk, sugar. Dinner: Lentil soup, fried steak, fried potatoes, white bread, butter (oleo), coffee, condensed milk, sugar.

Friday. Breakfast: Boiled rice, cheese, white bread, butter (oleo), fried beef, coffee, condensed milk, sugar. Dinner: Pea soup, salt fish and pot roast, boiled potatoes, canned vegetables served in juice that stood in cans, white bread, butter (oleo), coffee, condensed milk, sugar.

Saturday. Breakfast: Corned beef, cheese, fried potatoes, white bread, butter (oleo), coffee, condensed milk, sugar. Dinner: Potato soup, roast beef, boiled potatoes, white bread, butter (oleo), coffee, condensed milk, sugar.

Sunday. Breakfast: Beef stew, cheese, fried potatoes, white bread, butter (oleo), coffee, condensed milk, sugar. Dinner: Beef soup, pot roast, canned vegetables served in juice that stood in cans, boiled potatoes, white bread, butter (oleo).

"At 4 o'clock every afternoon the men were served a plate of Huntley & Palmer's fancy biscuits or sweet cakes with coffee, condensed milk and sugar."

Supper. "Evening meal either of fried steak, cold roast beef, corned beef, as beef stew with potatoes or cold roast beef with white bread, butter (oleo), coffee, condensed milk and sugar."

Does the menu sound familiar to you? It probably does because it is the diet civilized and affluent societies and countries generally consider necessary for "good health." The same menus are found in hotels, restaurants, airplanes and luxury liners. The sailors didn't dream of connecting their falling vitality and illness with what they ate. How many today even think of the foods they eat as possible detrimental health causes?

Not one of the officers fell ill to the extent suffered by the crew members. Why? We note that they received small quantities of fresh vegetables and fruits. This small ration was just enough to save them from the sickness of the crew. Do you see the wonderful building material found in natural foods—fruits and vegetables? Meet nature halfway, and she can do the rest. It is no credit to civilization that such a diet is common today. Where will it lead us? The prognosis is not encouraging.

Let me mention right here that hardening of the arteries creates devastating levels of blood pressure, increasing many times the risk of strokes.

Scientists tell us seawater carries the same chemical elements as the blood itself, but in much different proportions. I often wondered about how we could use the wonderful minerals in seawater to enrich our foods. Sometimes mineral-rich seaweed is used as fertilizer for crops. Diluted ocean water has also been used in trial studies.

Dr. Alexis Carrell kept a microsection of live cells from a chicken heart alive for about 30 years by feeding it casein in water. The casein fed the tissue and the water washed away the metabolic wastes. The tissue slice finally died when it was neglected for several days.

Today I am a great one for using iodine. Today I realize that a shortage of minerals is usually the beginning of every disease.

There's a lot being talked and thought about as far as the amount of sodium in foods is concerned. Truly the sodium that manufacturers and chemists are talking about is the sodium found in table salt. Table salt is processed at high heat to get rid of impurities, but we find in nature that sodium salts are always found in combination with other minerals, such as calcium, potassium, copper, magnesium, zinc and others. Sea salt contains a variety of minerals and is better for us than processed table salt.

I can almost tell the age of a cook in a restaurant. When the food is very salty, the cook is an older person. Older people, perhaps because of a lack of zinc to keep their taste buds working right, use more salt because it takes more before they can taste it. This is very dangerous.

The thyroid, which controls the metabolic rate, needs food iodine. Iodine, being water-soluble, tends to be lost when we use a lot of food cooked in water. The iodine is leached out of most cooked vegetables. This is one of the main reasons we should have iodine supplements of a natural type if we have a lot of cooked foods. Dulse or seaweed supplements are helpful. Most people eat too many cooked foods anyway and this always leaches away the iodine. Lack of iodine may reduce the metabolism and allow a person to gain excess weight. This is hard on the heart.

However, it isn't just a matter of using evaporated sea salt, because many times that has been heated through a high-heat process. It is best to use salt that comes from the ocean that has been sun dried. The more natural the process, the more compatible the food will be with the human body. We are dealing with trace minerals when taking salt in the form of sun-dried seawater.

Heart health is not just a matter of cutting out salt. We need a little salt, especially those who perspire a lot, such as women going through the change of life who are experiencing hot flashes. Get the proper kind of natural salt and add it to your foods only after it's cooked, not before. If you would like to investigate this further, you may write The Grain and Salt Society, P.O. Box DD, Magalia, CA 96954; telephone (916) 872-5800.

I find it very amusing to see that some people in restaurants start pouring salt on their food before they even taste it. This is a bad habit, and one that should be broken.

To the memory of my very good friend,
Abraham J. Rodriguez,
who recently passed away due to a sudden heart attack.

If You've Enjoyed Reading This Book . . .

Colostrum: Life's First Food—This book is full of fascinating surprises about a healing food that is "a new star on the health food horizon." It should be required reading for everyone interested in wellness and the reversal of disease. This food could be the solution to the health problems of the future.

Tissue Cleansing Through Bowel Management—Toxic-laden tissues can become a breeding ground for disease. Elimination organs, especially the bowel, must be properly taken care of to restore and maintain health. Learn Dr. Jensen's bowel management program. Discover the importance of balanced nutrition, dietary fiber and regular exercise. A cleansing treatment will bring back energy, regenerate tissues and allow food to let nature do its work in recovery.

Unfoldment of the Great Within—This new book presents some of the teachings of Dr. V.G. Rocine, together with Dr. Jensen's thoughts and philosophy. In learning ease of mind, we begin to push disease out of our bodies. We should know how to start a new life and new day to become a wiser, healthier and better person.

Goat Milk Magic—Goat milk promotes good health in many ways. One of its most remarkable features is that, for young and old alike who are prone to digestive distress of any kind, goat milk is the one food that stays down better than all other foods. The most sensitive stomach seems to welcome goat milk, and the most fatigued body seems to revive and thrive on it. This book should be in everyone's library.

Bee Well Bee Wise—Dr. Jensen is at his best in this fascinating book, sharing his insights on the blessings that hardworking honeybees have passed along to mankind. Pollen is a food substance, a highly-concentrated source of vitamins, minerals, enzymes, lecithin, hormone-like substances and a natural antibacterial substance, in a base of protein, carbohydrates and fatty acids.

Foods That Heal—In the first half of this book, Dr. Jensen focuses on the philosophy and ideas of Hippocrates, the brilliant work of Dr. V. G. Rocine, and concludes with a look at his own pioneering work in the field of nutrition. The second half is a nutritional guide to fruits and vegetables.

Juicing Therapy—Health through nature's most natural methods. How nature heals body organs and systems. Wonderful juice combination recipes. Juices for babies and children, soups, herbal green drinks, salad dressings. Special Analytical Food Guide chart.

Garlic Healing Powers—This book contains valuable information on how garlic plays such an important role as a member of the herbal kingdom. It includes garlic research, updates and uses as well as garlic recipes and other ways to enjoy garlic. You can also learn how to treat your family pets with the use of garlic.

Check at your local bookstore for information on Dr. Jensen's books and food products; if they cannot supply them, you may order directly from our office. For a *free* catalog of all his books and supplies, you may write to:

Dr. Bernard Jensen
24360 Old Wagon Road
Escondido, CA 92027